Pocket Reference
to Osteoporosis

T0073456

Serge Livio Ferrari • Christian Roux
Editors

Pocket Reference to Osteoporosis

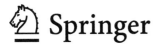 Springer

Editors
Serge Livio Ferrari
Division of Bone Diseases
Geneva University Hospital
and Faculty of Medicine
Geneva
Switzerland

Christian Roux
Department of Rheumatology
Paris Descartes University
Cochin Hospital
Paris
France

ISBN 978-3-319-26755-5   ISBN 978-3-319-26757-9   (eBook)
https://doi.org/10.1007/978-3-319-26757-9

Library of Congress Control Number: 2018964428

This Springer imprint is published by the registered company Springer Nature Switzerland AG
The registered company address is: Gewerbestrasse 11, 6330 Cham, Switzerland

Preface

Every few seconds, a patient is admitted to a hospital with a fragility fracture—namely, a fracture that occurred upon a minimal trauma, such as falling from one's own height. Whether treated surgically or conservatively, the risk of another fragility fracture is increased severalfold in such patients, unless the underlying cause is recognized and appropriately managed. The bulk of fragility fractures are caused by osteoporosis, a disease that affects nearly 300 million people worldwide and is a particular burden for aging populations. In most cases, diagnosing osteoporosis and evaluating fracture risk in due time, followed by appropriate treatment, could have prevented even the first fracture. Unfortunately, disorders of bone and mineral metabolism, including osteoporosis, are seldom taught to undergraduates. The resulting relative lack of knowledge has led to under-recognizing and undertreating the disease, with commonly less than 20% of osteoporotic patients being appropriately managed. A "crisis in osteoporosis" has therefore emerged that needs to be appropriately addressed. Whether a GP or a specialist in orthopaedics, endocrinology, rheumatology, gynaecology, or other specialties, every doctor should be aware of osteoporosis and be capable of managing the disease. This book has been written by some of the most prominent authorities in this field in order to provide the basic principles about osteoporosis in a practical way, in the hope of facilitating the diagnosis and treatment of devastating disease.

Geneva, Switzerland   Serge Livio Ferrari
Paris, France   Christian Roux

Contents

Contributors

Felicia Cosman, MD Helen Hayes Hospital, West Haverstraw, NY, USA

Serge Livio Ferrari, MD Division of Bone Diseases, Geneva University Hospital and Faculty of Medicine, Geneva, Switzerland

Piet Geusens, MD Department of Internal Medicine, Maastricht University Medical Center, Maastricht, The Netherlands

John A. Kanis, MD Center for Metabolic Bone Diseases, University of Sheffield Medical School, Sheffield, UK

Eugene V. McCloskey, MD Center for Metabolic Bone Diseases, University of Sheffield Medical School, Sheffield, UK

Michael R. McClung, MD Oregon Osteoporosis Center, Portland, OR, USA

Socrates E. Papapoulos, MD Center for Bone Quality, Leiden University Medical Center, Leiden, The Netherlands

René Rizzoli, MD Division of Bone Diseases, Geneva University Hospitals and Faculty of Medicine, Geneva, Switzerland

Christian Roux, MD Department of Rheumatology, Paris Descartes University, Cochin Hospital, Paris, Paris, France

Jopp van den Bergh, MD, PhD Department of Internal Medicine, Maastricht University Medical Center, Maastricht, The Netherlands

Chapter 1
Pathophysiology of Osteoporosis

Serge Livio Ferrari

1.1 Introduction

Bone is a dynamic tissue that is continuously removed and replaced (i.e., remodeled) in order to (1) ensure adaptation of the skeleton to weight-bearing (shape is function), (2) repair microdamages (cracks) that result from mechanical stresses, and (3) allow for mobilization of calcium from the skeleton in order to maintain serum calcium homeostasis [1]. Bone remodeling is initiated by the development and activation of osteoclasts, the bone-resorbing cell, which then release growth factors capable to activate osteoblasts, the bone-forming cell. The activities of bone removal and deposition are therefore coupled within each "bone multicellular unit" or BMU. After the completion of growth, the bone size and mineral content have reached its peak and will be maintained more or less unchanged during the adult life in the absence of pathophysiological conditions thanks to moderate levels of bone remodeling that are perfectly balanced between resorption and formation within each BMU. In addition, the skeleton continuously responds to mechanical stimuli resulting from both muscle contraction and weight-bearing, by directly stimulating

S. L. Ferrari (✉)
Division of Bone Diseases, Geneva University Hospital and Faculty of Medicine, Geneva, Switzerland
e-mail: serge.ferrari@unige.ch

© Springer Nature Switzerland AG 2019   1
S. L. Ferrari, C. Roux (eds.), *Pocket Reference to Osteoporosis*,
https://doi.org/10.1007/978-3-319-26757-9_1

bone formation (i.e., without prior resorption), a process known as bone modeling. This process in particular is responsible for the increased bone diameter and bone mass observed in physically active individuals, furthermore in athletes. It is controlled by osteocytes, which are terminally differentiated osteoblasts that have lost their capacity to form new bone but are entrenched in the bone and form a dense network of "sensing" cells capable to respond to mechanical stimuli, as well as to microdamages, and control both modeling and local remodeling processes [2].

1.2 The Pathophysiological Bases of Osteoporosis

Osteoporosis is a systemic skeletal disorder characterized by a decrease of bone mineral mass together with alterations of bone microstructure, particularly a reduction in the number and/or thinning of trabeculae with a loss of trabecular bridges, cortical thinning, and increased cortical porosity [3, 4]. These alterations are mainly the result of increased bone turnover triggered by the dramatic decline of estrogen levels in postmenopausal women. In men, aging and the decline in both testosterone and estrogen levels also play a role. At the cellular level, these endocrine disturbances lead to the activation of new BMUs that spread throughout cancellous and cortical bone surfaces. Moreover, within these foci of bone remodeling, a mismatch appears between the activity of osteoclasts and osteoblasts, resulting in a negative bone mineral balance (Fig. 1.1). Eventually, the senescence of osteocytes [5], together with the decline in physical functions with aging, may lead to a decrease of modeling-based bone formation.

In recent years, the key molecular mechanisms involved in the bone remodeling and modeling processes and the coupling between osteoblasts and osteoclasts have been elucidated. Among them, the Wnt/LRP5/beta-catenin

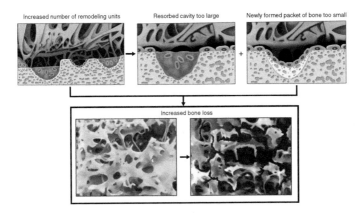

Increased number of remodeling units   Resorbed cavity too large   Newly formed packet of bone too small

Increased bone loss

FIGURE 1.1   Increased bone remodeling causes bone loss

canonical signaling pathway [6] and the RANKL/RANK/ OPG system [7] have emerged as playing essential roles in, respectively, bone-forming and bone resorption processes. In addition, the role of the immune system and the central nervous system on the regulation of bone turnover starts to be better appreciated. In turn, these remarkable progresses in the understanding of the pathophysiology of osteoporosis have delineated new targets for therapeutic developments.

1.3   The Role of Osteoclasts

The osteoclast (OC) is a bone tissue-specific multinucleated cell that differentiates from hematopoietic stem cells similar to those giving rise to monocyte/macrophage. Mature osteoclasts adhering to the bone surface both produce and secrete HCl, which acidifies and dissolves the bone mineral, and proteolytic enzymes, mainly metalloproteases and cathepsin K, which digest the bone matrix, releasing in the circulation-specific collagen fragments, such as CTx, which in turn are used as clinical markers of bone turnover.

Osteoclastogenesis is activated by a number of pro-inflammatory cytokines, including interleukin-1, interleukin-6, and TNF alpha, which can be expressed by both T cells in the bone marrow and bone cells themselves [8]. This explains why systemic inflammatory disorders, such as rheumatoid arthritis, cause accelerated bone loss. However the only two factors that are both necessary and sufficient to induce osteoclast differentiation are colony-stimulating factor-1 (CSF-1 or M-CSF) and receptor activator of nuclear factor kappa b (RANK) ligand (RANKL). The mature, multinucleated OC is further activated by RANKL binding to its receptor RANK.

To counteract the differentiation and activation of osteoclasts, osteoblasts/stromal cells also produce osteoprotegerin (OPG), a decoy receptor which binds RANKL, preventing its own binding to RANK (Fig. 1.2). Thereby, OPG negatively regulates osteoclastogenesis, promotes apoptosis of mature osteoclasts, and ultimately inhibits bone resorption [9]. Hence, it is not so much the absolute level of RANKL and OPG in the bone environment as much as the RANKL/OPG ratio that determines whether bone resorption will be stimulated or inhibited. In turn the discovery of RANKL/OPG led to the

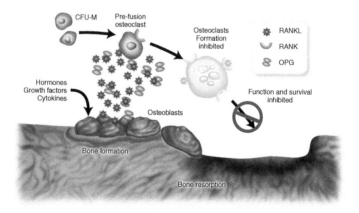

FIGURE 1.2 Osteoprotegerin (OPG), the natural antagonist of RANK ligand, inhibits osteoclastogenesis. (Adapted from Boyle et al. Nature. 2003;423:337–342.)

development of a human monoclonal antibody against RANKL, denosumab, to prevent osteolysis and bone loss [7] (see Chap. 5).

1.3.1   Control of Bone Resorption

Because the production of RANKL as well as other cytokines is downregulated by estrogen (Fig. 1.3), postmenopausal women suffer from an increased RANKL/OPG ratio that is a direct explanation for their accelerated bone turnover and bone loss [10].

Parathyroid hormone (PTH) is the other main hormone to be implicated in the pathogenesis of bone loss. Contrarily to estrogen receptors, the PTH/PTHrP receptor is expressed on osteoblasts rather than osteoclasts. PTH signaling in osteoblasts stimulates osteoclastogenesis, which is largely mediated by an increase in RANKL, concomitant decrease of OPG production, and therefore increase of the RANKL/OPG ratio [11]. This situation is reached when PTH levels are

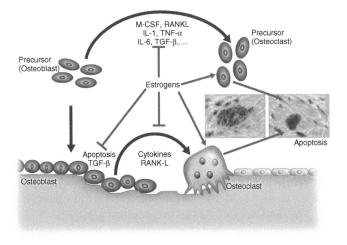

FIGURE 1.3 Estrogen controls cytokine production in bone and bone remodeling

elevated, such as during poor calcium intake, vitamin D deficiency, chronic renal failure, or in case of primary hyperparathyroidism due to pathophysiological growth of the parathyroid gland(s). In all these situations, increased PTH levels cause accelerated bone loss.

1.4   The Role of Osteoblasts

Osteoprogenitor cells arise from multipotential mesenchymal stem cells (MSCs) that give rise to a number of cell lineages including those for osteoblasts (OB), chondrocytes, and adipocytes [12]. Once osteoblasts are fully differentiated and become activated, they will fulfill their two major actions, namely, synthesize new bone matrix first (i.e., the osteoid), mainly constituted of type I collagen, then mineralize this osteoid by triggering the deposition of calcium-phosphate crystals named hydroxyapatite. This specific function involves tissue non-specific alkaline phosphatase (TNAP), which catalyzes the hydrolysis of phosphate esters at the osteoblast surface to provide a high phosphate concentration to initiate the bone mineralization process [13].

Whether or not osteoblastogenesis is impaired with aging remains uncertain. On one side, some in vitro experiments suggest that MSC proliferation and survival, as well as their differentiation into osteoblasts, are reduced from bone explants of elderly subjects compared to younger individuals. A reduced number of osteoblasts (and osteocytes; see below) and/or their impaired ability to synthesize new bone matrix in response to biomechanical stimulation has also been advocated as a potential mechanism for the reduced skeletal response to physical activity in the elderly (compared to growing and younger subjects) [14]. In turn, the aging skeleton seems to accumulate more fat cells resulting from the preferential differentiation of MSCs into adipocytes in the bone marrow [15].

1.4.1   Control of Bone Formation

Several signaling molecules play major roles in controlling differentiation toward the osteoblastic lineage. These include insulin-like growth factor 1 (IGF-1) and other growth factors that stimulate bone formation, as well as cytokines, particularly interleukin-6, which exert negative effects. Hence decreased levels of IGF-1, which has also been related to poor protein intake, may contribute to decreased bone mass with aging [16].

The essential role of wingless (Wnt) canonical signaling on bone formation was understood when loss-of-function mutations in the low-density lipoprotein receptor-related protein 5 (LRP5), a Wnt receptor expressed in bone cells, were discovered to cause the osteoporosis-pseudoglioma syndrome (OPPG), an autosomal recessive disorder characterized by extremely low BMD and skeletal fragility [17]. On the opposite, gain-of-function mutation in LRP5 causes high bone mass (HBM) phenotypes and diverse sclerosing bone dysplasias. Furthermore, mutations in or near the *SOST* gene, coding for sclerostin, were found responsible for the rare sclerosing bone dysplasias, sclerosteosis, and van Buchem disease type 1 [18, 19]. Similar to LRP5 HBM mutations, SOST mutations are characterized by a marked increase in bone mass. Expression of the *SOST* gene product, sclerostin, is restricted to osteocytes in adults and was revealed as an osteocyte-specific negative regulator of bone formation [20, 21] (Fig. 1.4). Production of sclerostin by osteocytes is rapidly decreased by mechanical loading and by PTH [22, 23]. Whether sclerostin expression is increased, or inappropriate,

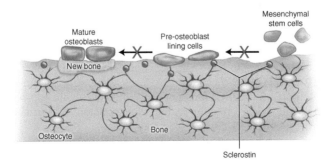

FIGURE 1.4 Sclerostin produced by osteocytes inhibits bone formation

with aging and contributes directly to osteoporosis remains unclear. Nevertheless its discovery has allowed the development of neutralizing monoclonal antibodies with remarkable bone-forming properties [24] (see Chap. 9).

1.5   Conclusion

The loss of bone mineral mass and the microstructural alterations that fragilize bone, leading to osteoporosis, result from complex cellular and molecular mechanisms. Those are represented by increased osteoclast numbers and activity driven primarily by RANK ligand and a relatively weaker bone-forming response by osteoblasts, which are negatively controlled by sclerostin from osteocytes. In turn, these mechanisms have become the target for osteoporosis treatment.

References

1. Hadjidakis DJ, Androulakis II. Bone remodeling. Ann N Y Acad Sci. 2006;1092:385–96.
2. Bonewald LF. The amazing osteocyte. J Bone Miner Res. 2011;26(2):229–38.
3. Seeman E, Delmas PD. Bone quality--the material and structural basis of bone strength and fragility. N Engl J Med. 2006;354(21):2250–61.
4. Zebaze RM, Ghasem-Zadeh A, Bohte A, et al. Intracortical remodelling and porosity in the distal radius and post-mortem femurs of women: a cross-sectional study. Lancet. 2010;375(9727):1729–36.
5. Farr JN, Fraser DG, Wang H, et al. Identification of senescent cells in the bone microenvironment. J Bone Miner Res. 2016;31(11):1920–9.
6. Baron R, Rawadi G. Targeting the Wnt/beta-catenin pathway to regulate bone formation in the adult skeleton. Endocrinology. 2007;148(6):2635–43.
7. Kearns AE, Khosla S, Kostenuik PJ. Receptor activator of nuclear factor kappaB ligand and osteoprotegerin regulation of bone remodeling in health and disease. Endocr Rev. 2008;29(2):155–92.

8. Bruzzaniti A, Baron R. Molecular regulation of osteoclast activity. Rev Endocr Metab Disord. 2006;7(1–2):123–39.
9. Simonet WS, Lacey DL, Dunstan CR, et al. Osteoprotegerin: a novel secreted protein involved in the regulation of bone density. Cell. 1997;89(2):309–19.
10. Eghbali-Fatourechi G, Khosla S, Sanyal A, Boyle WJ, Lacey DL, Riggs BL. Role of RANK ligand in mediating increased bone resorption in early postmenopausal women. J Clin Invest. 2003;111(8):1221–30.
11. Ma YL, Cain RL, Halladay DL, et al. Catabolic effects of continuous human PTH (1--38) in vivo is associated with sustained stimulation of RANKL and inhibition of osteoprotegerin and gene-associated bone formation. Endocrinology. 2001;142(9):4047–54.
12. Heino TJ, Hentunen TA. Differentiation of osteoblasts and osteocytes from mesenchymal stem cells. Curr Stem Cell Res Ther. 2008;3(2):131–45.
13. Murshed M, Harmey D, Millan JL, McKee MD, Karsenty G. Unique coexpression in osteoblasts of broadly expressed genes accounts for the spatial restriction of ECM mineralization to bone. Genes Dev. 2005;19(9):1093–104.
14. Seeman E. Loading and bone fragility. J Bone Miner Metab. 2005;23(Suppl):23–9.
15. Duque G. Bone and fat connection in aging bone. Curr Opin Rheumatol. 2008;20(4):429–34.
16. Bonjour JP, Schurch MA, Chevalley T, Ammann P, Rizzoli R. Protein intake, IGF-1 and osteoporosis. Osteoporos Int. 1997;7(3):S36–42.
17. Gong Y, Slee RB, Fukai N, et al. LDL receptor-related protein 5 (LRP5) affects bone accrual and eye development. Cell. 2001;107(4):513–23.
18. Brunkow ME, Gardner JC, Van Ness J, et al. Bone dysplasia sclerosteosis results from loss of the SOST gene product, a novel cystine knot-containing protein. Am J Hum Genet. 2001;68(3):577–89.
19. Staehling-Hampton K, Proll S, Paeper BW, et al. A 52-kb deletion in the SOST-MEOX1 intergenic region on 17q12-q21 is associated with van Buchem disease in the Dutch population. Am J Med Genet. 2002;110(2):144–52.
20. van Bezooijen RL, Roelen BA, Visser A, et al. Sclerostin is an osteocyte-expressed negative regulator of bone formation, but not a classical BMP antagonist. J Exp Med. 2004;199(6):805–14.

21. Poole KE, van Bezooijen RL, Loveridge N, et al. Sclerostin is a delayed secreted product of osteocytes that inhibits bone formation. FASEB J. 2005;19(13):1842–4.
22. Bellido T, Ali AA, Gubrij I, et al. Chronic elevation of parathyroid hormone in mice reduces expression of sclerostin by osteocytes: a novel mechanism for hormonal control of osteoblastogenesis. Endocrinology. 2005;146(11):4577–83.
23. Keller H, Kneissel M. SOST is a target gene for PTH in bone. Bone. 2005;37(2):148–58.
24. Ke HZ, Richards WG, Li X, Ominsky MS. Sclerostin and dickkopf-1 as therapeutic targets in bone diseases. Endocr Rev. 2012;33:747.

Chapter 2
Diagnosis and Clinical Aspects of Osteoporosis

John A. Kanis

2.1 Introduction

The internationally agreed description of osteoporosis is "a systemic skeletal disease characterized by low bone mass and microarchitectural deterioration of bone tissue with a consequent increase in bone fragility and susceptibility to fracture" [1]. This description captures the notion that low bone mass is an important component of the risk of fracture but that other abnormalities occur in the skeleton that contribute to skeletal fragility. Thus, ideally, clinical assessment of the skeleton should capture all these aspects of fracture risk. At present, however, the assessment of bone mineral is the only aspect that can be readily measured in clinical practice, and it now forms the cornerstone for the description of osteoporosis.

2.2 Diagnosing Osteoporosis

Although diagnosis of the disease relies on the quantitative assessment of bone mineral density, which is a major determinant of bone strength, the clinical significance of osteoporosis

J. A. Kanis (✉)
Center for Metabolic Bone Diseases, University of Sheffield Medical School, Sheffield, UK
e-mail: w.j.pontefract@shef.ac.uk

© Springer Nature Switzerland AG 2019
S. L. Ferrari, C. Roux (eds.), *Pocket Reference to Osteoporosis*,
https://doi.org/10.1007/978-3-319-26757-9_2

lies in the fractures that arise. In this respect, there are some analogies with other multifactorial chronic diseases. For example, hypertension is diagnosed on the basis of blood pressure, whereas an important clinical consequence of hypertension is stroke.

Because a variety of non-skeletal factors contribute to fracture risk, the diagnosis of osteoporosis by the use of bone mineral density (BMD) measurements is at the same time an assessment of a risk factor for the clinical outcome of fracture. For these reasons, there is a distinction to be made between the use of BMD for diagnosis and for risk assessment [2].

Bone mineral density is most often described as a T- or Z-score, both of which are units of standard deviation (SD). The T-score describes the number of SDs by which the BMD in an individual differs from the mean value expected in young healthy individuals (Fig. 2.1). The operational definition of osteoporosis is based on the T-score for BMD [3] assessed at the femoral neck and is defined as a value for BMD 2.5 SD or more below the young female adult mean (T-score less than or equal to −2.5 SD) [4]. The Z-score describes the number of SDs by which the BMD in an individual differs from the mean value expected for age and sex. It is mostly used in children and adolescents. The recommended reference range by the for calculating the T-score is the National Health and Nutrition Examination Survey (NHANES) III reference database for femoral neck measurements in Caucasian women aged 20–29 years [5]. The diagnostic criteria for men use the same female reference range as that for women. In clinical practice osteoporosis is commonly defined as a T-score applied to other sites (e.g., lumbar spine).

2.3   Osteoporotic Fractures

An osteoporotic fracture describes a fracture event arising from trauma that in a healthy individual would not give rise to fracture. A widely adopted approach is to consider fractures

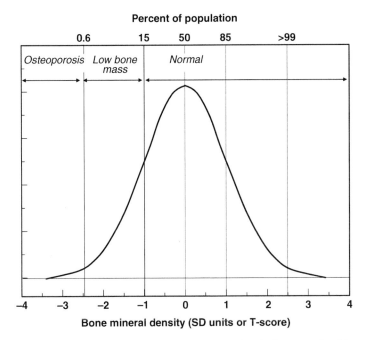

FIGURE 2.1 The distribution of bone mineral density in young healthy women in standard deviation units and threshold values for osteoporosis and low bone mass (osteopenia). *SD* standard deviation

from low energy trauma as being osteoporotic. "Low energy" is defined as a fall from a standing height or less. However, osteoporotic patients more frequently sustain fractures after "high-energy" trauma than their non-osteoporotic counterparts [6]. An approach increasingly used is to characterize fracture sites as osteoporotic when they are associated with low bone mass and their incidence rises with age after the age of 50 years [7]. The most common fractures defined in this way are those at the hip, spine, and forearm (Fig. 2.2), but many other fractures after the age of 50 years are related at least in part to low BMD and should be regarded as osteoporotic. These include fractures of the humerus, ribs, tibia (in women but not including ankle fractures), pelvis, and other

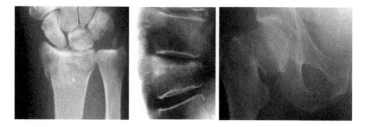

FIGURE 2.2 Typical sites of osteoporotic fracture: wrist (left), spine (center), and hip (right)

femoral fractures. Under this schema, the fracture sites that would be excluded include those at the ankle, hands, and feet, including the digits, skull and face, and kneecap.

2.3.1 Hip Fracture

Hip fracture is the most serious osteoporotic fracture. Most hip fractures follow a fall from the standing position. About one third of elderly individuals fall annually, and 5% will sustain a fracture with 1% suffering a hip fracture [8]. Hip fracture is painful and nearly always necessitates hospitalization.

The two main hip fracture types, cervical or trochanteric, have a somewhat different natural history and treatment. In many countries both fracture types occur with equal frequency, though the average age of patients with trochanteric fractures is approximately 5 years older than for cervical fractures. Displaced cervical fractures have a high incidence of malunion and osteonecrosis following internal fixation, and the prognosis is improved with hip replacement. Trochanteric hip fractures appear to heal normally after adequate surgical management. For both fracture types, there is a high degree of morbidity and appreciable mortality that depend in part on the age, the treatment given, and the associated morbidity. Up to 20% of patients die in the first year following hip fracture, mostly as a result of serious

Annual Incidence (rate/1,000)

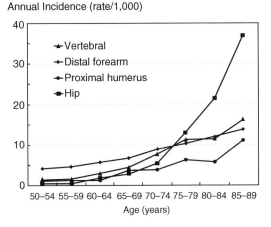

FIGURE 2.3 Incidence (rate/1000 per annum) by age of fractures at the sites shown in women from Malmo, Sweden. Vertebral fractures are those coming to clinical attention [Drawn from data in 12]

underlying medical conditions, and less than half of survivors regain the level of function that they had prior to the hip fracture [9, 10].

Incidence rates for hip fracture increase exponentially with age in both men and women (Fig. 2.3). Rates for men at any age are about half that in women. There is a remarkable heterogeneity in the age-adjusted and sex-adjusted incidence for hip fracture in various regions of the world which varies more than tenfold [11]. The highest incidence rates have been observed in Northern Europe.

2.3.2   Vertebral Fracture

Vertebral fracture is the most difficult osteoporosis-related fracture to define. The problem arises in part because the diagnosis is made on a change in the shape of the vertebral body and a substantial proportion of vertebral deformities are clinically silent or not attributable to osteoporosis. About one in three vertebral deformities reaches immediate clinical attention through either back pain, height loss, or other functional impairment [12]. Scheuermann's disease (osteochondritis) and vertebral osteoarthritis are common disorders that give rise to deformities not attributable to osteoporosis.

The deformities that result from osteoporotic fracture are classified as a crush fracture (involving compression of the entire vertebral body), a wedge fracture (in which there is anterior height loss), and biconcavity (where there is relative maintenance of the anterior and posterior heights with central compression of the end-plate regions).

The vast majority of vertebral fractures are a result of moderate or minimal trauma. Falls account for only about one third of new clinical vertebral fractures, and most are associated instead with other activities such as lifting or changing position.

Incidence rates can be expressed as the incidence of vertebral deformity (morphometric fractures) or the incidence of clinically overt fractures (clinical vertebral fractures) [13]. The incidence of vertebral morphometric deformities, as with other osteoporotic fractures, is greater in women than in men and rises with age. The age-related increase is less steep than that of hip fractures (see Fig. 2.3), and the variation between countries is less marked. The incidence of clinically evident vertebral fractures is 20–40% that of morphometric fractures [12].

2.3.3   Distal Forearm Fracture

The most common distal forearm fracture is Colles' fracture associated with dorsal angulation and displacement of the distal fragment of the radius, often accompanied by a fracture of the ulna styloid process. The cause of fracture is usually a fall on the outstretched hand. Although fractures of the wrist cause less morbidity than hip fractures, are rarely fatal, and seldom require hospitalization, the consequences are often underestimated. Fractures are painful, usually require one or more reductions, and need 4–6 weeks in plaster. Approximately 1% of patients with a forearm fracture become dependent as a result of the fracture, but nearly half report only fair or poor functional outcome at 6 months [8, 14].

Forearm fractures display a different pattern of incidence from that of hip or spine fractures. In many countries, rates increase linearly in women between the ages of 40 and 65 years and then stabilize. In other countries, incidence rises progressively with age (see Fig. 3.3). Forearm fractures are much less frequent in men; the incidence is commonly constant between the ages of 20 and 80 years, and where this rises, it does so at a much slower rate than in women.

2.3.4   All Fractures

A majority of fractures in patients aged 50 years or more are attributable to osteoporosis. The incidence rates of proximal humeral, pelvic, and proximal tibial fractures rise steeply with age and are greater among women than among men. At the age of 50 years, rib, vertebral, and forearm fractures are the most commonly found fractures in men, whereas in women the most common fractures comprise distal forearm, vertebral, rib, and proximal humeral fractures. Over the age of 85 years, hip fracture is the most frequent fracture among men and women but still accounts for only approximately one third of all osteoporotic fractures [7].

2.4   Burden of Disease

There are different ways of expressing the burden of disease. From an individual perspective, the likelihood of fracture from the age of 50 years is a useful metric (Table 2.1). The remaining lifetime probability in women at the menopause of a fracture at any one of these sites exceeds that of breast cancer (approximately 12%), and the likelihood of a fracture at any of these sites is 40% or more in Western Europe [15], a figure close to the probability of coronary heart disease.

TABLE 2.1 Remaining lifetime probability of a major osteoporotic fracture at the age of 50 and 80 years in men and women from Sweden [15]

	At 50 years		At 80 years	
Site	Men	Women	Men	Women
Forearm	4.6	20.8	1.6	8.9
Hip	10.7	22.9	9.1	49.3
Spine	8.3	15.1	4.7	8.7
Humerus	4.1	12.9	2.5	7.7
Any of these	22.4	46.4	15.3	31.7

With kind permission from Springer Science and Business Media

The number of new fractures in 2010 in the EU was estimated at 3.5 million, comprising approximately 620,000 hip fractures, 520,000 vertebral fractures, 560,000 forearm fractures, and 1,800,000 other fractures [8]. Thus, hip, vertebral, forearm, and "other fractures" accounted for 18%, 15%, 16%, and 51% of all fractures, respectively. Two thirds of all incident fractures occurred in women. Osteoporotic fractures accounted for €37.4 billion in direct costs in the 27 EU countries [16, 17].

2.5   Conclusion

The high societal and personal costs of osteoporosis pose challenges to public health and physicians, particularly since most patients with osteoporosis remain untreated. Moreover, age is an important risk factor for fractures, and the elderly population is projected to increase in the majority of countries, which will increase the burden of fracture. Projections for Europe indicate that the number of osteoporotic fractures will increase by 28% from 3.5 million in 2010 to 4.5 million in 2025 [16].

The operational definition of osteoporosis, based on spine or hip BMD T-scores evaluated by DXA scans, has proven a practical tool in identifying affected individuals at higher risk of fragility fractures. However, because the pathophysiological definition of osteoporosis is more complex and includes dimensions that are not fully appreciated by DXA, a majority of fragility fractures still occurs in osteopenic subjects.

References

1. Anonymous. Consensus Development Conference. Diagnosis, prophylaxis and treatment of osteoporosis. Am J Med. 1993;94:646–50.
2. Kanis JA, McCloskey EV, Johansson H, et al. European guidance for the diagnosis and management of osteoporosis in postmenopausal women. Osteoporos Int. 2013;24:23–57.
3. [No authors listed]. Assessment of fracture risk and its application to screening for postmenopausal osteoporosis. World Health Organ Tech Rep Ser. 1994;843:1–129.
4. Kanis JA, McCloskey EV, Johansson H, Oden A, Melton LJ 3rd, Khaltaev N. A reference standard for the description of osteoporosis. Bone. 2008;42:467–75.
5. Looker AC, Wahner HW, Dunn WL, ct al. Updated data on proximal femur bone mineral levels of US adults. Osteoporos Int. 1998;8:468–86.
6. Sanders KM, Pasco JA, Ugoni AM, et al. The exclusion of high trauma fractures may underestimate the prevalence of bone fragility fractures in the community: the Geelong Osteoporosis Study. J Bone Miner Res. 1998;13:1337–42.
7. Kanis JA, Oden A, Johnell O, Jonsson B, de Laet C, Dawson A. The burden of osteoporotic fractures: a method for setting intervention thresholds. Osteoporos Int. 2001;12:417–27.
8. Kanis JA on behalf of the World Health Organization Scientific Group. Assessment of osteoporosis at the primary healthcare level. Technical Report. WHO Collaborating Centre for Metabolic Bone Diseases, University of Sheffield, UK, 2008. http://www.shef.ac.uk/FRAX/pdfs/WHO_Technical_Report.pdf. Accessed 5 Jan 2016.
9. Poór G, Atkinson EJ, O'Fallon WM, Melton LJ 3rd. Determinants of reduced survival following hip fractures in men. Clin Orthop Rel Res. 1995;319:260–5.
10. Melton LJ 3rd. Adverse outcomes of osteoporotic fractures in the general population. J Bone Miner Res. 2003;18:1139–41.

11. Kanis JA, Odén A, McCloskey EV, Johansson H, Wahl D, Cooper C, IOF Working Group on Epidemiology and Quality of Life. A systematic review of hip fracture incidence and probability of fracture worldwide. Osteoporos Int. 2012;23:2239–56.
12. Kanis JA, Johnell O, Oden A, et al. Risk and burden of vertebral fractures in Sweden. Osteoporos Int. 2004;15:20–6.
13. O'Neill TW, Cockerill W, Matthis C, et al. Back pain, disability and prevalent vertebral fracture: a prospective study. Osteoporos Int. 2004;15:760–5.
14. Kaukonen JP, Karaharju EO, Porras M, Lüthje P, Jakobsson A. Functional recovery after fractures of the distal forearm: analysis of radiographic and other factors affecting the outcome. Ann Chir Gynaecol. 1988;77:27–31.
15. Kanis JA, Johnell O, Oden A, et al. Long-term risk of osteoporotic fracture in Malmo. Osteoporos Int. 2000;11:669–74.
16. Hernlund E, Svedbom A, Ivergård M, et al. Osteoporosis in the European Union: medical management, epidemiology and economic burden. A report prepared in collaboration with the International Osteoporosis Foundation (IOF) and the European Federation of Pharmaceutical Industry Associations (EFPIA). Arch Osteoporos. 2013;8:136.
17. Svedbom A, Hernlund E, Ivergård M, et al. Osteoporosis in the European Union: a compendium of country-specific reports. Arch Osteoporos. 2013;8:137.

Chapter 3
Evaluation of Fracture Risk

Eugene V. McCloskey

3.1 Introduction

The World Health Organization (WHO) diagnostic criterion for osteoporosis, launched in 1994 [1], was based on the bone mineral density (BMD) T-score (<-2.5) and is still used in many healthcare systems as a necessary requirement for reimbursement of osteoporosis therapies that reduce fracture risk. However, as implied by this chapter title, and indeed the definition of osteoporosis itself (see Chap. 2), there is more to the assessment of fracture risk than simply the identification of BMD-defined osteoporosis.

3.2 Non-invasive Skeletal Assessments

3.2.1 Measurements of Bone Mass

Dual-energy X-ray absorptiometry (DXA) is by far the most commonly used assessment of bone mass and has been validated for the assessment of fracture risk in many studies [2].

E. V. McCloskey (✉)
Center for Metabolic Bone Diseases, University of Sheffield Medical School, Sheffield, UK
e-mail: e.v.mccloskey@sheffield.ac.uk

© Springer Nature Switzerland AG 2019
S. L. Ferrari, C. Roux (eds.), *Pocket Reference to Osteoporosis*,
https://doi.org/10.1007/978-3-319-26757-9_3

DXA scanners measure the attenuation through the body of X-ray beams with two different photon energies [3] with regard to two reference materials, namely, bone mineral (hydroxyapatite) and soft tissue (defined within a reference area adjacent to the bone region of interest). Edge detection software is used to find the bone outline at skeletal sites, most commonly the lumbar spine and proximal femur. The technique is fast and uses a low radiation dose. Several manufacturers provide DXA equipment with subtle but occasionally important differences in voltages used, filtering mechanisms, edge detection, and soft tissue thickness adjustments. For these reasons, care needs to be taken when comparing results from the same patients scanned across different makes of equipment – ideally, patients should be scanned on the same equipment over time, where possible. The main indication for the measurement of BMD by DXA is the presence of risk factors, such as prior fracture, family history of fracture, causes of secondary osteoporosis (e.g. rheumatoid arthritis, glucocorticoid use, etc.), and lifestyle factors with only small variation across healthcare systems. Some clinical guidelines now recommend the formal assessment of fracture risk prior to BMD assessment (see below) [4].

Quantitative computed tomography (QCT) is a potential alternative to DXA but largely remains a research tool. It offers the advantage of providing a true volumetric density as well as an assessment of bone microstructure [3]. The X-ray dose is substantially higher than DXA although recent developments targeting the peripheral skeleton (tibia and radius/ulna) provide lower exposures. In QCT, a reference phantom of known composition is scanned together with the patient to permit expression of the results in calcium hydroxyapatite equivalent BMD.

Quantitative ultrasound (QUS) is also a common tool used in the assessment of bone mass (it may also capture bone structure, but its contribution to the clinical utility of QUS appears marginal). The heel is the only validated skeletal site for the clinical use of QUS and predicts fragility fracture in postmenopausal women (hip, vertebral, and global fracture risk) and older men, independently of axial BMD [5]. Axial DXA at the spine and femur remains the preferred measurement for making therapeutic decisions and should be used if possible.

3.2.2   Measurements of Bone Structure

Non-invasive imaging can assess bone macrostructure and microstructure. Lateral imaging of the spine using DXA is now a well-established method for vertebral fracture assessment (VFA), so that a single device can capture two well-established risk factors for fracture (BMD and the presence or absence of vertebral fracture; Fig. 3.1). VFA can be undertaken in patients at higher risk of having a prevalent vertebral fracture, for example, in older individuals, patients with historical or measured height loss, self-reported prior fracture, and long-term glucocorticoid therapy [6].

FIGURE 3.1 Vertebral fracture assessment image from a dual-energy X-ray absorptiometry scanner of the thoracic and lumbar spine showing a vertebral fracture at the thoraco-lumbar junction

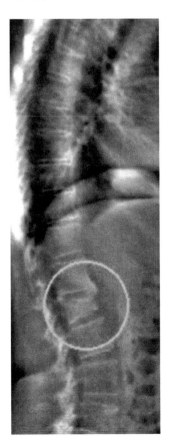

More recently, a third clinically applicable, DXA-based assessment has been developed, namely, the trabecular bone score (TBS). TBS is a grey-level textural measurement originally derived from lumbar spine DXA images that appears to be an index of bone microarchitecture. Prospective studies have shown that TBS predicts fracture in postmenopausal women and older men, independently of BMD [7]. DXA can also be used to examine macrostructural parameters such as hip shape, buckling index, and femoral neck length although these are not commonly used in clinical practice. More detailed microstructural imaging using high-resolution peripheral QCT is available as a research tool [8].

3.2.3   Measurements of Bone Turnover

Despite the knowledge that high bone turnover is often detrimental and that inhibitors of bone turnover are beneficial, the uptake of bone turnover markers (BTM) in clinical use has been slowed by concerns about their variability and inadequate quality control [9]. BTM predict fracture risk, though weakly, and treatment-induced changes in specific markers account for a substantial proportion of fracture risk reduction. More recent, better validated markers for bone formation, such as serum aminoterminal propeptide of type I collagen (PINP), and bone resorption, serum carboxy (C)-terminal telopeptide (CTX), are increasingly available and are being incorporated into monitoring algorithms of osteoporosis therapies. Uncertainties over their clinical use continue to be resolved through the development and adoption of international reference standards.

3.3   Assessment of Fracture Risk

The principal difficulty with the use of BMD alone for risk assessment is that BMD has high specificity but low sensitivity for future fractures. Thus, the majority of hip and other osteoporotic fractures will occur in individuals with BMD

TABLE 3.1 Summary of the characteristics of three available fracture risk assessment tools

	Garvan	Qfracture	FRAX
Externally validated	Yes (a few countries)	Yes (UK only)	Yes
Calibrated	No	No	Yes
Applicability	Unknown	UK	64 countries
Falls as an input	Yes	Yes	No
BMD as an input variable	Yes	No	Yes
Prior fracture as an input	Yes	Yes	Yes
Family history as an input	No	Yes	Yes
Output	Incidence	Incidence	Probability
Treatment response assessed	No	No	Yes

values above the osteoporosis threshold [1]. In clinical practice, many still use the multiple skeletal site approach (lowest T-score of the spine, hip, or femoral neck) in the belief that this improves the sensitivity of the technique but without recognizing that this does not enhance the performance of the test in terms of predictive value (the gain in sensitivity is offset by a loss of specificity).

In the past 20 years, a great deal of research has taken place to identify factors other than BMD that contribute to fracture risk. Examples include age, sex, a prior fracture, a family history of fracture, and lifestyle risk factors such as physical inactivity and smoking. Some of these risk factors are partially or wholly independent of BMD; they can therefore enhance the information provided by BMD alone or, conversely, if strongly correlated with BMD can be used for fracture risk assessment in the absence of BMD tests [10].

Several fracture prediction tools are available and increasingly used in clinical practice. All have limitations (Table 3.1), but all perform better than the simple use of a single risk factor (e.g. BMD) alone.

Only the FRAX® tool has been calibrated to rates of fracture and mortality per individual country and has been shown to identify a risk amenable to currently available treatments. It is a computer-based algorithm (http://www.shef.ac.uk/FRAX) that provides models for the assessment of 10-year fracture probability in men and women using easily obtained clinical risk factors, with or without femoral neck BMD (Fig. 3.2).

FRAX calculates the 10-year probability of major osteoporotic fractures (hip, clinical spine, humerus, or wrist fracture) and the 10-year probability of hip fracture alone. At present, 68 FRAX models are available for 64 countries. In the absence of a FRAX model for a particular country, a surrogate country should be chosen, based on the likelihood that it is representative of the index country. In addition to the web-based calculator, the tool is also available in other formats including being available on densitometers and

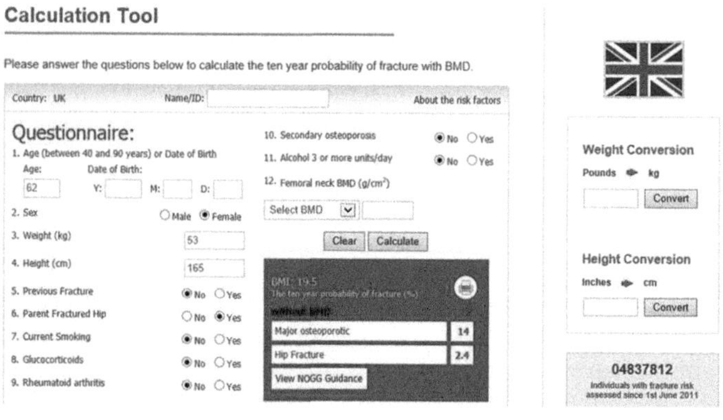

FIGURE 3.2 Screenshot of the UK FRAX® calculation tool showing the risk factors and outputs of 10-year probabilities of major osteoporotic and hip fractures

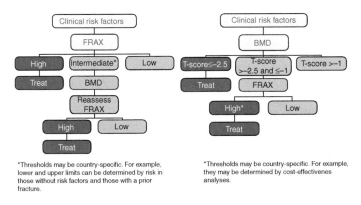

*Thresholds may be country-specific. For example, lower and upper limits can be determined by risk in those without risk factors and those with a prior fracture.

*Thresholds may be country-specific. For example, they may be determined by cost-effectivenes analyses.

FIGURE 3.3 Approaches to the use of fracture risk assessment using FRAX® in different guidelines depending on DXA availability

smartphones. FRAX is incorporated into a large number of assessment guidelines [11], some of which recommend the use of FRAX prior to BMD measurement (e.g. in the UK and Europe) [12, 13] and some which recommend BMD first (e.g. the USA; Fig. 3.3) [14], largely determined by the availability of DXA equipment. A recent study testing the UK approach, based on FRAX hip fracture probabilities, has shown a 28% reduction in hip fractures [15].

3.4   Conclusion

The advent of risk assessment algorithms indicates that prevention of fractures is better targeted on the basis of fracture probability using multiple risk factors rather than BMD alone. Increasingly, guidelines are implementing risk-based assessment and intervention into routine clinical practice. Notwithstanding, diagnostic criteria remain of value in quantifying the burden of disease, the development of strategies to combat osteoporosis, and at least for the immediate future, as a criterion for reimbursement in many healthcare systems.

References

1. [No authors listed]. Assessment of fracture risk and its application to screening for postmenopausal osteoporosis. Report of a WHO Study Group. World Health Organ Tech Rep Ser. 1994;843:1–129.
2. Johnell O, et al. Predictive value of BMD for hip and other fractures. J Bone Miner Res. 2005;20(7):1185–94.
3. Genant HK, et al. Noninvasive assessment of bone mineral and structure: state of the art. J Bone Miner Res. 1996;11(6):707–30.
4. National Institute for Health and Care Excellence NICE Clinical Guideline 146. Osteoporosis: assessing the risk of fragility fracture. 2012. DOI: guidance.nice.org.uk/CG146.
5. Knapp KM. Quantitative ultrasound and bone health. Salud Publica Mex. 2009;51(Suppl 1):S18–24.
6. International Society for Clinical Densitometry, Official Positions 2015 ISCD Combined. 2015.
7. Silva BC, et al. Trabecular bone score: a noninvasive analytical method based upon the DXA image. J Bone Miner Res. 2014;29(3):518–30.
8. Boutroy S, et al. In vivo assessment of trabecular bone microarchitecture by high-resolution peripheral quantitative computed tomography. J Clin Endocrinol Metab. 2005;90(12):6508–15.
9. Vasikaran S, et al. International Osteoporosis Foundation and International Federation of Clinical Chemistry and Laboratory Medicine position on bone marker standards in osteoporosis. Clin Chem Lab Med. 2011;49(8):1271–4.
10. Kanis JA. on behalf of the WHO Scientific Group, Assessment of osteoporosis at the primary health-care level. Technical Report. 2008, WHO Collaborating Centre, University of Sheffield, UK: Sheffield.
11. Kanis JA, et al. SCOPE: a scorecard for osteoporosis in Europe. Arch Osteoporos. 2013;8(1–2):144.
12. Kanis JA, et al. European guidance for the diagnosis and management of osteoporosis in postmenopausal women. Osteoporos Int. 2013;24(1):23–57.
13. Compston J, et al. Diagnosis and management of osteoporosis in postmenopausal women and older men in the UK: National Osteoporosis Guideline Group (NOGG) update 2013. Maturitas. 2013;75(4):392–6.

14. Dawson-Hughes B, et al. Implications of absolute fracture risk assessment for osteoporosis practice guidelines in the USA. Osteoporos Int. 2008;19(4):449–58.
15. Shepstone L, et al. Screening in the community to reduce fractures in older women (SCOOP): a randomised controlled trial. Lancet. 2018;391(10122):741–7.

Chapter 4
Prevention of Osteoporosis and Fragility Fractures

René Rizzoli

4.1 Introduction

A fracture represents a structural failure of the bone whereby the forces applied to the bone exceed its load-bearing capacity. Therefore, besides bone geometry, mass, density, microstructure, and material level properties, the direction and magnitude of the applied load also determine whether a bone will fracture. Almost all fractures, even those qualified as "low-trauma" fractures, occur as the result of some injury, for instance, a fall from standing height or bending forward to lift heavy objects for vertebral fracture. While available pharmacological intervention is primarily aimed at restoring bone strength (i.e., reducing bone fragility) by altering bone turnover and/or material level properties, a variety of preventive measures for osteoporotic fractures are capable of influencing both components of fracture risk: mechanical overload, for example, falls, and mechanical incompetence, such as osteoporosis (Fig. 4.1).

R. Rizzoli (✉)
Division of Bone Diseases, Geneva University Hospitals and
Faculty of Medicine, Geneva, Switzerland
e-mail: rene.rizzoli@unige.ch

© Springer Nature Switzerland AG 2019   31
S. L. Ferrari, C. Roux (eds.), *Pocket Reference to Osteoporosis*,
https://doi.org/10.1007/978-3-319-26757-9_4

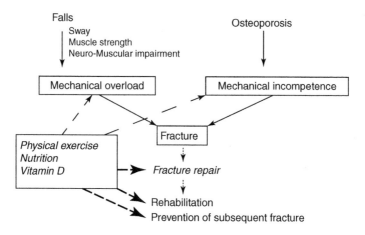

FIGURE 4.1 Prevention of osteoporotic fracture by physical exercise, nutrition (calcium, protein), and vitamin D

4.2   Physical Activity

Immobilization is an important cause of bone loss [1]. Immobilized patients may lose as much bone in a week when confined to bed as they would otherwise lose in a year. At the tissue level, immobilization results in a negative balance, the amount of bone resorbed being greater than that formed. At the cellular level, immobilization results in an increased osteoclastic resorption associated with a decrease in osteoblastic formation. The amount of weight-bearing exercise that is optimal for skeletal health in patients with osteoporosis is not known, but exercise forms an integral component of its management [2, 3]. Physiotherapy is an important component of rehabilitation after fracture [4]. At all times, increased muscle strength may prevent falls by improving confidence and coordination and contribute to reducing fracture risk by maintaining bone mass through a stimulation of bone formation and a decrease of bone resorption [5].

Mixed loading exercise appears to be effective to reduce bone loss in postmenopausal women [6–8] and in men [9]. Some prevention of hip fracture by physical activity has been consistently reported [10]. Jumping on one leg daily during 12 months is associated with an increased cortical thickness of the femoral neck [10].

The potential side effects and limitations of physical activity in osteoporotic patients have been reviewed, as reported in 39 intervention studies (Table 4.1) [11].

Both aerobic activity and resistance training are of benefit to older people. Resistance exercise training is a stimulus for muscle protein synthesis and appears to be beneficial to rebuild muscle mass, strength, and performance in the elderly [5]. Dietary proteins following physical exercises magnify de novo muscle protein synthesis [12, 13]. The American Heart Association and the American College of Sports Medicine encourage older adults to complete 30–60 min of moderate intensity aerobic exercise per day (150–300 min/week) or 20–30 min of vigorous intensity exercise per day (75–150 min/week) [14]. For healthy older adults, exercise of 10–15 min per session with eight repetitions for each muscle group is a reasonable goal.

TABLE 4.1   Physical activity in osteoporotic patients

Patients at high risk of fracture (with prevalent fracture or with glucocorticoid therapy): avoid trunk flexion exercise; however, trunk extension exercise and abdominal stabilization exercise are safe (level 2, grade A).

Patients recovering from hip fracture: weight-bearing exercises are recommended from day 18 (level 2, grade A).

Patients with osteoporosis: aerobic physical activity and progressive resistance training are safe (level 2, grade A). They should avoid powerful twisting movements of the trunk (level 3, grade C).

Patients with spinal cord injury (without recent fracture): progressive lower limb resistance training or body-weight-supported treadmill (level 2, grade A). Avoid maximal strength testing, for instance, by electrical stimulation (level 3, grade C).

Level of evidence (1, RCTs; 2, RCTs with limitation or very convincing observational studies; 3, observational studies; 4, anecdotal evidence) and recommendations grades (A, strong; B, intermediate; C, weak)

4.3   Prevention of Falls

The risk of falling increases with age. Most falls in elderly are due to intrinsic and extrinsic or environmental factors (Table 4.2) [15].

4.3.1   Intrinsic Factors

The risk of falling increases with the number of disabilities. Impairments of gait, mobility, and balance have been the most consistently identified risk factors for falls and fall-related injuries [15]. Thus, the risk of falling increases with reduced visual acuity or diminished sensory perception of the lower extremities. Chronic illnesses such as various neurological disorders, heart diseases, stroke, urinary incontinence, depression, and impaired cognitive functions increase the risk of falling. Medications such as hypnotics, antidepressants, or sedatives are associated with falls [16].

4.3.2   Environmental (Extrinsic) Risk Factors

Potential hazards that can be found in the home include slippery floors, unstable furniture, and insufficient lighting.

TABLE 4.2 Risk factors associated with falls

1. Impaired mobility, disability
2. Impaired gait and balance
3. Neuromuscular or musculoskeletal disorders
4. Age
5. Impaired vision
6. Neurological, heart disorders
7. History of falls
8. Medication
9. Cognitive impairment

Modifiable factors such as correcting decreased visual acuity [17], reducing consumption of medication that alters alertness and balance, and improving the home environment (slippery floors, obstacles, insufficient lighting, and handrails) are important measures aimed at preventing falls [15, 18, 19]. Recently, a multitask music-based training such as Jaques-Dalcroze eurhythmic exercises has been shown to reduce gait and balance variability and lower fracture incidence [20, 21]. Some studies, although not all, have reported fall risk reduction in the elderly that practice Tai Chi [22]. Large trials have shown that it is possible to reduce falls [18, 23], and meta-analyses have concluded that reducing falls can be associated with a lower fracture risk [24].

4.4   Nutrition

There is a high prevalence of calcium, protein, and vitamin D deficiency in the elderly population [25–28], which plays a significant role in osteoporosis, sarcopenia, and in fracture risk [29–31]. Malnutrition appears to be more severe in patients with hip fracture than in the general aging population. Mechanisms for alterations of protein use in older persons are inadequate intake of protein, reduced ability to use available protein (e.g., anabolic resistance and tissue redistribution of amino acids), and a greater need for protein (e.g., in inflammatory diseases). Dietary proteins have a direct effect on key regulatory proteins and growth factors involved in muscle metabolism, such as mammalian target of rapamycin (mTOR) and insulin-like growth factor-1 (IGF-1) [5]. Branched-chain amino acids lead to activation of mTOR, and aromatic amino acids (which are particularly prevalent in dairy protein) lead to increased IGF-1 resulting in greater muscle mass and strength. Recommended dietary allowance for protein in adults is 0.8 g of protein per kilogram of body weight each day (g/kg BW/d). A low dietary intake of protein (0.45 g/kg BW) in elderly healthy women, a level quite common in patients presenting with hip fracture, is associated with a reduction in plasma IGF-1 levels and in skeletal muscle fiber atrophy [32].

A low protein intake could be particularly detrimental since it alters the conservation of muscle and bone integrity with aging [25, 29]. Protein malnutrition can favor the occurrence of hip fracture by increasing the propensity to fall as a result of muscle weakness and of impairment in movement coordination, by affecting protective mechanisms, and thus by reducing the energy required to fracture an osteoporotic proximal femur and/or by decreasing bone mass [31]. In addition to lower IGF-1, a low protein intake is associated with decreased intestinal absorption of calcium and secondary hyperparathyroidism [33].

There is a positive correlation between bone mineral mass and spontaneous protein intake in women [34], with a meta-analysis showing that 1–4% of bone mineral density (BMD) variance could be explained by protein intakes. In a prospective study carried out on more than 40,000 women in Iowa, higher protein intake was associated with a reduced risk of hip fracture [35].

Whereas a gradual decline in caloric intake with age can be considered as an appropriate adjustment to the progressive reduction in energy expenditure, the parallel reduction in protein intake may be detrimental for maintaining the integrity and function of several organs or systems, including skeletal muscle and bone [25]. Intakes of at least 1 g/kg body weight of protein are recommended in the general management of patients with osteoporosis [36] and even 1.2 g/kg in the elderly [29, 36, 37].

A state of malnutrition at admission in elderly patients with hip fracture followed by an inadequate food intake during hospital stay can adversely influence their clinical outcome. Intervention studies using a simple oral dietary preparation that normalizes protein intake can improve the clinical outcome after hip fracture [25, 38] and reduce the length of stay for rehabilitation in hospital [39]. Thus, sufficient protein intakes are necessary to maintain the function of the musculoskeletal system and to decrease the medical complications that occur after an osteoporotic fracture [39].

4.4.1   Calcium and Vitamin D

At every stage of life, adequate dietary intakes of key bone nutrients such as calcium and vitamin D contribute to bone health and reduce the risk of osteoporosis and fracture later in life [30, 40]. Dietary sources of calcium are the preferred option, and calcium supplementation should only be targeted to those who do not get sufficient calcium from their diet and who are at high risk for osteoporosis. Calcium-rich foods such as dairy products contain additional nutrients that may also contribute to bone health [41].

The recommended nutrient intakes (RNI) are at least 1000 mg of calcium and 800 international units (IU) of vitamin D per day in men and women over the age of 60 years [27, 42]. As dairy is the main source of calcium, calcium- and vitamin D-fortified dairy products (such as yogurt and milk) providing around 40% of the RNI of calcium (400 mg) and 200 IU of vitamin D per portion are valuable options, likely to improve long-term adherence [41, 42]. When pharmacological calcium supplements are needed, they should be taken with a meal to improve tolerance and increase calcium absorption.

Most randomized controlled trial evidence for the efficacy of interventions is based on co-administration of the agent with calcium and vitamin D supplements [40]. Calcium and vitamin D supplements decrease secondary hyperparathyroidism and reduce the risk of proximal femur fracture, particularly in the elderly living in nursing homes. Intakes of at least 1000 mg/day of calcium and 800 IU of vitamin D can be recommended in the general management of patients with osteoporosis [37, 42].

A recent meta-analysis has concluded that calcium supplements without co-administered vitamin D were associated with an increased risk of myocardial infarction [43]. Cardiovascular outcomes were not primary endpoints in any of the studies, and this analysis is the subject of controversy. Large long-term observational studies have not confirmed this hypothesis [44, 45]. There was no increased risk when calcium was of dietary origin [43].

Vitamin D has both skeletal and extra-skeletal benefits [29]. The potential effect of vitamin D on skeletal muscle strength is receiving attention. Vitamin D supplements alone may reduce the risk of fracture and of falling provided the daily dose of vitamin D is greater than 700 IU [30]. In contrast, studies with large annual doses of vitamin D have reported an increased risk of falls and hip fracture [46]. Thus, a yearly regimen of vitamin D high-dose supplementation should be avoided.

4.5   Conclusion

For the management of osteoporosis, protein intake of 1.0–1.2 g/kg BW/d, calcium intake of 1000 mg/day, and vitamin D supplements of 800–1000 IU/d are associated with higher muscle strength and improved bone health [37]. The positive effect of physical activity on muscle protein synthesis and function is augmented by protein intake [12, 13].

References

1. Vico L, Collet P, Guignandon A, et al. Effects of long-term microgravity exposure on cancellous and cortical weight-bearing bones of cosmonauts. Lancet. 2000;355:1607–11.
2. Bonaiuti D, Shea B, Iovine R, et al. Exercise for preventing and treating osteoporosis in postmenopausal women. Cochrane Database Syst Rev. 2002:CD000333.
3. Howe TE, Shea B, Dawson LJ, et al. Exercise for preventing and treating osteoporosis in postmenopausal women. Cochrane Database Syst Rev. 2002:CD000333.
4. Auais MA, Eilayyan O, Mayo NE. Extended exercise rehabilitation after hip fracture improves patients' physical function: a systematic review and meta-analysis. Phys Ther. 2012;92:1437–51.
5. Girgis CM. Integrated therapies for osteoporosis and sarcopenia: from signaling pathways to clinical trials. Calcif Tissue Int. 2015;96:243–55.

6. Martyn-St James M, Carroll S. Meta-analysis of walking for preservation of bone mineral density in postmenopausal women. Bone. 2008;43:521–31.

7. Martyn-St James M, Carroll S. A meta-analysis of impact exercise on postmenopausal bone loss: the case for mixed loading exercise programmes. Br J Sports Med. 2009;43:898–908.

8. Kelley GA, Kelley KS, Kohrt WM. Effects of ground and joint reaction force exercise on lumbar spine and femoral neck bone mineral density in postmenopausal women: a meta-analysis of randomized controlled trials. BMC Musculoskeletal Disord. 2012;13:177.

9. Kelley GA, Kelley KS, Kohrt WM. Exercise and bone mineral density in men: a meta-analysis of randomized controlled trials. Bone. 2013;53:103–11.

10. Karlsson MK, Nordqvist A, Karlsson C. Physical activity, muscle function, falls and fractures. Food Nutr Res. 2008;52:1920.

11. Chilibeck PD, Vatanparast H, Cornish SM, Abeysekara S, Charlesworth S. Evidence-based risk assessment and recommendations for physical activity: arthritis, osteoporosis, and low back pain. Appl Physiol Nutr Metab. 2011;36(Suppl 1):S49–79.

12. Cermak NM, Res PT, de Groot LC, Saris WH, van Loon LJ. Protein supplementation augments the adaptive response of skeletal muscle to resistance-type exercise training: a meta-analysis. Am J Clin Nutr. 2012;96:1454–64.

13. Finger D, Goltz FR, Umpierre D, Meyer E, Rosa LH, Schneider CD. Effects of protein supplementation in older adults undergoing resistance training: a systematic review and meta-analysis. Sports Med. 2015;45:245–55.

14. Nelson ME, Rejeski WJ, Blair SN, et al. Physical activity and public health in older adults: recommendation from the American College of Sports Medicine and the American Heart Association. Med Sci Sports Exerc. 2007;39:1435–45.

15. Panel on Prevention of Falls in Older Persons, American Geriatrics Society and British Geriatrics Society. Summary of the Updated American Geriatrics Society/British Geriatrics Society clinical practice guideline for prevention of falls in older persons. J Am Geriatr Soc. 2011;59:148–57.

16. Woolcott JC, Richardson KJ, Wiens MO, et al. Meta-analysis of the impact of 9 medication classes on falls in elderly persons. Arch Intern Med. 2009;169:1952–60.

17. Harwood RH, Foss AJ, Osborn F, Gregson RM, Zaman A, Masud T. Falls and health status in elderly women following

first eye cataract surgery: a randomised controlled trial. Br J Opthalmol. 2005;89:53–9.

18. Gillespie LD, Robertson MC, Gillespie WJ, et al. Interventions for preventing falls in older people living in the community. Cochrane Database Syst Rev. 2012;9:CD007146.

19. Sherrington C, Tiedemann A. Physiotherapy in the prevention of falls in older people. J Physiother. 2015;61:54–60.

20. Trombetti A, Hars M, Herrmann FR, Kressig RW, Ferrari S, Rizzoli R. Effect of music-based multitask training on gait, balance, and fall risk in elderly people: a randomized controlled trial. Arch Intern Med. 2011;171:525–33.

21. Hars M, Herrmann FR, Fielding RA, Reid KF, Rizzoli R, Trombetti A. Long-term exercise in older adults: 4-year outcomes of music-based multitask training. Calcif Tissue Int. 2014;95:393–404.

22. Low S, Ang LW, Goh KS, Chew SK. A systematic review of the effectiveness of Tai Chi on fall reduction among the elderly. Arch Gerontol Geriatr. 2009;48:325–31.

23. Oliver D, Connelly JB, Victor CR, et al. Strategies to prevent falls and fractures in hospitals and care homes and effect of cognitive impairment: systematic review and meta-analyses. BMJ. 2007;334:82.

24. El-Khoury F, Cassou B, Charles MA, Dargent-Molina P. The effect of fall prevention exercise programmes on fall induced injuries in community dwelling older adults: systematic review and meta-analysis of randomised controlled trials. BMJ. 2013;347:f6234.

25. Rizzoli R. Nutritional aspects of bone health. Best Pract Res Clin Endocrinol Metab. 2014;28:795–808.

26. Bischoff-Ferrari HA, Kiel DP, Dawson-Hughes B, et al. Dietary calcium and serum 25-hydroxyvitamin D status in relation to BMD among U.S. adults. J Bone Miner Res. 2009;24:935–42.

27. Ross AC, Manson JE, Abrams SA, et al. The 2011 report on dietary reference intakes for calcium and vitamin D from the Institute of Medicine: what clinicians need to know. J Clin Endocrinol Metab. 2011;96:53–8.

28. Mithal A, Wahl DA, Bonjour JP, et al. Global vitamin D status and determinants of hypovitaminosis D. Osteoporosis Int. 2009;20:1807–20.

29. Rizzoli R, Stevenson JC, Bauer JM, et al. The role of dietary protein and vitamin D in maintaining musculoskeletal health in postmenopausal women: a consensus statement from the European

Society for Clinical and Economic Aspects of Osteoporosis and Osteoarthritis (ESCEO). Maturitas. 2014;79:122–32.

30. Bischoff-Ferrari HA, Willett WC, Orav EJ, et al. A pooled analysis of vitamin D dose requirements for fracture prevention. N Engl J Med. 2012;367:40–9.

31. Gaffney-Stomberg E, Insogna KL, Rodriguez NR, Kerstetter JE. Increasing dietary protein requirements in elderly people for optimal muscle and bone health. J Am Geriatr Soc. 2009; 57:1073–9.

32. Castaneda C, Gordon PL, Fielding RA, Evans WJ, Crim MC. Marginal protein intake results in reduced plasma IGF-I levels and skeletal muscle fiber atrophy in elderly women. J Nutr Health Aging. 2000;4:85–90.

33. Kerstetter JE, O'Brien KO, Caseria DM, Wall DE, Insogna KL. The impact of dietary protein on calcium absorption and kinetic measures of bone turnover in women. J Clin Endocrinol Metab. 2005;90:26–31.

34. Darling AL, Millward DJ, Torgerson DJ, Hewitt CE, Lanham-New SA. Dietary protein and bone health: a systematic review and meta-analysis. Am J Clin Nutr. 2009;90:1674–92.

35. Munger RG, Cerhan JR, Chiu BC. Prospective study of dietary protein intake and risk of hip fracture in postmenopausal women. Am J Clin Nutr. 1999;69:147–52.

36. Bauer J, Biolo G, Cederholm T, et al. Evidence-based recommendations for optimal dietary protein intake in older people: a position paper from the PROT-AGE Study Group. J Am Med Dir Assoc. 2013;14:542–59.

37. Rizzoli R, Branco J, Brandi ML, et al. Management of osteoporosis of the oldest old. Osteoporosis Int. 2014;25:2507–29.

38. Feldblum I, German L, Castel H, Harman-Boehm I, Shahar DR. Individualized nutritional intervention during and after hospitalization: the nutrition intervention study clinical trial. J Am Geriatr Soc. 2011;59:10–7.

39. Schurch MA, Rizzoli R, Slosman D, Vadas L, Vergnaud P, Bonjour JP. Protein supplements increase serum insulin-like growth factor-I levels and attenuate proximal femur bone loss in patients with recent hip fracture. A randomized, double-blind, placebo-controlled trial. Ann Intern Med. 1998;128:801–9.

40. Tang BM, Eslick GD, Nowson C, Smith C, Bensoussan A. Use of calcium or calcium in combination with vitamin D supplementation to prevent fractures and bone loss in people aged 50 years and older: a meta-analysis. Lancet. 2007;370:657–66.

41. Rizzoli R. Dairy products, yogurts, and bone health. Am J Clin Nutr. 2014;99:1256S–62S.
42. Kanis JA, McCloskey EV, Johansson H, et al. European guidance for the diagnosis and management of osteoporosis in postmenopausal women. Osteoporosis Int. 2013;24:23–57.
43. Bolland MJ, Avenell A, Baron JA, et al. Effect of calcium supplements on risk of myocardial infarction and cardiovascular events: meta-analysis. BMJ. 2013;c3691:341.
44. Prentice RL, Pettinger MB, Jackson RD, et al. Health risks and benefits from calcium and vitamin D supplementation: Women's Health Initiative clinical trial and cohort study. Osteoporosis Int. 2013;24:567–80.
45. Paik JM, Curhan GC, Sun Q, et al. Calcium supplement intake and risk of cardiovascular disease in women. Osteoporosis Int. 2014;25:2047–56.
46. Sanders KM, Stuart AL, Williamson EJ, et al. Annual high-dose oral vitamin D and falls and fractures in older women: a randomized controlled trial. JAMA. 2010;303:1815–22.

Chapter 5
Efficacy and Safety of Osteoporosis Treatment

Michael R. McClung

5.1 Introduction

For postmenopausal women with osteoporosis, pharmacological therapy compliments adequate nutrition, regular physical activity, and, when appropriate, strategies to prevent falls, alleviate pain, and optimize function. The objective of drug therapy is to reduce the incidence of serious fragility fractures that can impair function, degrade quality of life, and even increase the risk of death. Several drugs with different mechanisms of action are available for clinical use. This chapter will review the effectiveness, important safety issues, and practical considerations in choosing among the most important treatment options. Salmon calcitonin (limited evidence of efficacy and no longer available in Europe) and strontium ranelate (modest evidence of efficacy, significant restrictions on use in Europe, and never available in the United States) will not be discussed.

M. R. McClung (✉)
Oregon Osteoporosis Center, Portland, OR, USA
e-mail: mmcclung@orost.com

© Springer Nature Switzerland AG 2019
S. L. Ferrari, C. Roux (eds.), *Pocket Reference to Osteoporosis*,
https://doi.org/10.1007/978-3-319-26757-9_5

5.2   Bisphosphonates

Nitrogen-containing bisphosphonates, congeners of pyrophosphate, are the most studied and most commonly used drugs for the treatment of osteoporosis. Four members of this class of drugs are in clinical use (Tables 5.1 and 5.2).

These organic compounds bind tightly but variably to bone matrix. Upon endocytosis into osteoclasts, important synthetic pathways are interrupted, resulting in decreased osteoclast function, reduction in bone resorption, and, secondarily, decreased bone formation [10]. Drug not bound to the bone is rapidly excreted and unmetabolized via the urinary tract. Poor absorption of orally administered bisphosphonates, blunted even more in the presence of food, requires strict oral dosing rules: the drug should be taken after an overnight fast at least 30–60 min before food or beverages other than water.

After 3 years of treatment, bone mineral density (BMD) increases of 5–7% and 1.6–5% are noted in the spine and femoral neck, respectively [1, 2, 4, 5]. BMD in the proximal femur does not increase further with treatment after 5 years (Fig. 5.1).

Reductions in vertebral fracture risk of 60–70% are observed within the first year of treatment. Significant reductions in non-vertebral fractures (20–30%) and hip fractures (40–50%) have been reported with each drug except ibandronate [1–3, 5]. The effects of treatment on indices of bone remodeling persist as long as treatment is administered without evidence of pharmacological resistance [11–13]. The reduction in fracture risk also persists but does not improve with long-term therapy. Upon stopping treatment after several years, bone turnover markers return to baseline values within 12 months of stopping risedronate but remain below baseline for several years upon stopping alendronate or zoledronic acid [14–16]. Protection from vertebral fracture is at least partially lost within 3–5 years after stopping alendronate or zoledronic acid [15, 16].

Bisphosphonates have been well-tolerated in clinical trials. In clinical practice, upper gastrointestinal (GI) intolerance

TABLE 5.1 Effects of therapies on fracture risk in postmenopausal women with osteoporosis

Drug	References	Years	Vertebral fracture			Non-vertebral fracture			Hip fracture		
			Incidence (%)		Relative risk reduction	Incidence (%)		Relative risk reduction	Incidence (%)		Relative risk reduction
			Placebo	Treatment		Placebo	Treatment		Placebo	Treatment	
Alendronate	[1]	3	15	8	47%	14.7	11.9	20%	2.2	1.1	51%
Risedronate	[2, 3]	3	16.3	11.8	41%	8.4	5.2	40%	3.2	1.9	40%
Ibandronate	[4]	3	9.6	4.7	62%	8.2	9.1	NS	Not reported		
Zoledronic acid	[5]	3	10.9	3.3	70%	10.8	8	25%	2.5	1.4	41%
Denosumab	[6]	3	7.2	2.3	68%	8.0	6.5	20%	1.2	0.7	40%
Teriparatide	[7]	1.6	14	5	65%	9.7	6.3	35%	Not reported		
Raloxifene	[8]	3	4.5[a]	2.3[a]	50%[a]	9.3	8.5	NS	0.7	0.8	NS
			21.2[b]	14.7[b]	30%[b]						
Bazedoxifene	[9]	3	4.1	2.3	42%	6.3	5.7	NS	Not reported		

Because data are from individual clinical trials, direct comparisons of efficacy cannot be made

[a]In patients without prior vertebral fractures

[b]In patients with prior vertebral fractures; *NS* not significant

TABLE 5.2 Osteoporosis drugs: dosing, contraindications, and precautions

Drug	Dose	Route of administration	Contraindications[a]	Important warnings or precautions[a]
Bisphosphonates				
Alendronate	10 mg daily 70 mg weekly	Oral	Hypocalcemia Esophageal stricture or dysfunction	Not recommended in patients with eGFR <30–35 cc/min
Risedronate	5 mg daily 35 mg weekly 150 mg monthly	Oral	Inability to remain upright after dosing patients at increased risk of aspiration	
Ibandronate	150 mg monthly 3 mg Q 3 months	Oral Intravenous		
Zoledronic acid	5 mg Q 12 months	Intravenous	Hypersensitivity Hypocalcemia eGFR <35 cc/min	Severe incapacitating bone, joint, and/or muscle pain may occur

Denosumab	60 mg Q 6 months	Subcutaneous	Hypersensitivity Hypocalcemia Pregnancy	–
Teriparatide	20 ugm daily	Subcutaneous	Hypersensitivity	At risk for osteosarcoma[b] Active or recent urolithiasis Patients with bone metastases, history of skeletal malignancies, metabolic bone diseases other than osteoporosis, or hypercalcemic disorders
Estrogen agonists/antagonists				
Raloxifene	60 mg daily	Oral	Active or past history of venous thromboembolism Pregnancy Nursing mothers	Hepatic impairment Hypertriglyceridemia Risk of death from stroke in patients at increased risk for major coronary events

(continued)

Table 5.2 (continued)

Drug	Dose	Route of administration	Contraindications[a]	Important warnings or precautions[a]
Bazedoxifene	20 mg daily	Oral	Hypersensitivity Active or past history of venous thromboembolic events Women of child-bearing potential Unexplained uterine bleeding Evidence of endometrial cancer	Hypertriglyceridemia Hepatic or severe renal impairment

[a]According to the US Food and Drug Administration prescribing information for each drug except European Medicines Agency prescribing information for bazedoxifene
[b]Patients with Paget's disease of bone, pediatric and young adult patients with open epiphyses, and patients with prior external beam or implant radiation involving the skeleton

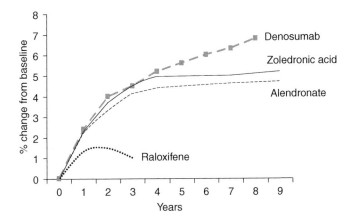

FIGURE 5.1 Percentage change in bone mineral density (BMD) from baseline in response to treatment with raloxifene [8], alendronate [1], zoledronic acid (femoral neck BMD [5]), and denosumab (total hip BMD [6])

occurs with oral dosing, and flu-like symptoms occur with initial intravenous doses [17]. Osteonecrosis of the jaw occurs commonly in patients receiving high doses of bisphosphonates for treatment of cancer-related bone disease but occurs very rarely with osteoporosis doses. Femoral shaft fractures with atypical features are observed with long-term bisphosphonate therapy, and the risk appears to increase with longer duration of treatment. In patients with osteoporosis, the reduction in the incidence of vertebral and hip fracture far exceeds the risk of atypical femoral fracture, even after 10 years of treatment. Based on the limited evidence available, temporary interruption of therapy is recommended after 3–5 years in patients at modest risk for fractures, while the benefit/risk ratio remains favorable for patients at high risk, at least up to 10 years [18]. Rare cases of hypersensitivity and of inflammatory eye disease have been reported. Concerning signals about atrial fibrillation with intravenous zoledronic acid and esophageal cancer with oral bisphosphonates have not been confirmed [17]. No impairment of fracture healing has been observed in clinical studies. Hypocalcemia upon starting therapy can occur in patients with vitamin D deficiency, and adequate intake of calcium and vitamin D should be assured before treatment begins [19–22]. Mortality after hip fracture is reduced with alendronate or zoledronic acid therapy [23, 24].

Few patients with impaired renal function were included in clinical trials, and no renal safety issues were noted in those studies [25]. In clinical practice, renal failure has been reported with intravenous zoledronic acid therapy, and this drug is contraindicated in patients with glomerular filtration rate (GFR) <35 mL per minute (Table 5.2) [22]. Alendronate and risedronate are not recommended in patients with estimated GFR <30 or 35 mL/min [20, 21].

5.3   Estrogen Agonist/Antagonists

Estrogen agonist/antagonists (previously selective estrogen receptor modulators or SERMs) are weak activators of the estrogen receptor in skeletal tissue while inhibiting the effects of estrogen in reproductive tissues. Raloxifene is approved for treating women with postmenopausal osteoporosis in both North America and Europe, while bazedoxifene is approved for the same indication only in Europe. Treatment with both drugs induces modest reduction in markers of bone turnover and increases in bone mineral density [8, 9]. In women with postmenopausal osteoporosis, raloxifene for 3 years decreased the incidence of vertebral fracture by 30–50% [8]. No effect was observed on the risk of non-vertebral or hip fracture. In a head-to-head study, bazedoxifene and raloxifene were similar in their effects on fracture risk [9]. By antagonizing estrogen in breast tissue, raloxifene decreases the risk of invasive breast cancer by 70% [26]. No effect of bazedoxifene on breast cancer risk was observed [9]. Both drugs are associated with an estrogen-like two- to three-fold increase in the risk of venous thrombotic events [27, 28]. In women at high risk for cardiovascular disease, raloxifene was associated with a twofold increase in the risk of death from stroke although the incidence of stroke or cardiac arrhythmias was not increased with therapy [29].

5.4   Denosumab

Denosumab, a fully human monoclonal antibody, binds specifically to receptor activator of nuclear factor kappa-B (RANK) ligand. By inactivating RANK ligand, the proliferation and activation of osteoclasts are inhibited, resulting in substantial reduction in bone turnover. Subcutaneous dosing with 60 mg provides substantial inhibition of bone turnover for 6 months [30]. BMD progressively increases with therapy, achieving after average increments of 21.7% and 9.2% in dual-energy X-ray absorptiometry (DXA) measurements of the spine and hip, respectively, over 10 years [31]. In the FREEDOM pivotal fracture trial, the risk of vertebral, hip, and spinal fracture was reduced by 68%, 40%, and 20%, respectively, with denosumab therapy over 3 years [6]. These effects on fracture risk were observed as early as 12 months and appear to persist for at least 10 years. Switching from a bisphosphonate to denosumab results in slightly greater gains in BMD than if the patient remains on the bisphosphonate [32].

No major safety issues have been observed in clinical trials. A modest increase frequency of skin rash and cellulitis, not associated with injection site, was noted during the first 3 years of the FREEDOM study [6]. The incidence of these skin affects did not increase with therapy over 10 years and was not increased in patients who had received placebo during years 1–3 of the FREEDOM study but who then took denosumab during years 4–10 in the extension study [31]. A theoretical risk of immune dysfunction has not been observed. Rare cases of atypical femoral fracture and osteonecrosis of the jaw were observed in the FREEDOM extension study, but the number of cases is much too low to know if this is truly a consequence of treatment or if the risk of this possible side effect is related to the duration of treatment [31]. Rare cases of anaphylaxis, usually following the first dose, have been reported [33].

As with all potent anti-remodeling agents, hypocalcemia can occur when denosumab treatment is initiated, especially in patients who have vitamin D deficiency, severe renal impairment, or hypoparathyroidism [33]. Adequate intake of calcium and vitamin D should be provided before treatment begins.

Because denosumab is not cleared by the kidney and is not nephrotoxic, its use is not contraindicated in patients with severe renal impairment. The effect of denosumab on BMD and vertebral fracture risk is similar in patients with chronic kidney disease stage III and IV compared to patients with normal renal function [34]. The benefits and risks of denosumab therapy in patients on dialysis have not been evaluated thoroughly.

There is no limit to the duration of denosumab therapy. Upon discontinuing denosumab, markers of bone turnover return to or rise above baseline values within 9 months of the last dose, BMD gradually returns toward baseline values, and protection from vertebral fracture risk is lost within a few months [35, 36]. Multiple and severe vertebral fractures have been reported in patients who stop denosumab, and transition to another anti-remodeling drug should be considered [7].

5.5   Teriparatide

Teriparatide (recombinant human parathyroid hormone 1–34), when administered daily by subcutaneous injection, activates bone remodeling with bone formation exceeding bone resorption leading to progressive increases in BMD and improved trabecular microarchitecture [37]. Estimated strength of cortical bone (proximal femur or hip region) increases despite an increase, at least transiently, in cortical porosity [38].

In the Pivotal Fracture Trial, women with established osteoporosis therapy were treated with teriparatide 20 μg or 40 μg daily for an average of 19 months [39]. With the 20 μg daily dose, spine and hip BMD by DXA increased by 9.1% and 5%, respectively. This was associated with a 65% reduction in the incidence of vertebral fracture and a 35% decrease in non-vertebral fracture risk. Too few hip fractures occurred in the study to evaluate the effect of therapy on hip fracture risk. In postmenopausal women with previous vertebral fractures, teriparatide was more effective than risedronate in reducing the risk of vertebral fractures within 12 months and of non-vertebral fracture within 24 months [40].

Adverse effects, usually mild and self-limited, included hypercalcemia, nausea, and light-headedness. Because high-dose, lifelong teriparatide therapy in rats induced a dose-related increase in osteosarcoma, teriparatide is contraindicated in patients at risk for osteosarcoma including children and adolescents (Table 5.1) [38]. Therapy is also limited by regulatory authorities to 18 months in Europe and to 24 months in the United States.

5.6   Choosing Among Therapies

In the absence of contraindications, bisphosphonates and denosumab are first-line therapies for all women with post-menopausal osteoporosis. For patients with upper GI tract abnormalities (e.g., gastrectomy, celiac disease, and Crohn's disease) or in whom concern exists about adherence to therapy, intravenous zoledronic acid or subcutaneous denosumab ensures absorption and compliance. Denosumab is an appropriate choice in patients who cannot take bisphosphonates because of impaired renal function. Raloxifene and (in Europe) bazedoxifene are excellent options in younger post-menopausal women with osteoporosis who are at high risk for spinal fracture but low risk for hip fracture, especially in those with risk factors for breast cancer. Teriparatide is appropriate for patients at high risk for vertebral fracture, including patients with previous vertebral fractures and low spine BMD. It is also used in patients who are intolerant of or who have poor or inadequate responses to anti-resorptive drugs.

5.7   Conclusion

Several drugs are effective in reducing the risks of important fractures. The classes of drugs differ in their mechanisms of action, potency, and side effect profiles, but among drugs within a particular class, the effects appear to be similar. Serious side effects are possible with each class of drug, but these risks can be reduced by avoiding treatment in patients at risk for a side effect and educating patients to notify their physician upon the appearance of symptoms of possible side effects such as calf pain with raloxifene or thigh pain with bisphosphonates. When patients at high risk of fracture are treated, the benefits of fracture reduction far outweigh the risk of a serious adverse event.

References

1. Black DM, Cummings SR, Karpf DB, et al. Randomised trial of effect of alendronate on risk of fracture in women with existing vertebral fractures. Lancet. 1996;348:1535–41.
2. Harris ST, Watts NB, Genant HK, et al. Effects of risedronate treatment on vertebral and nonvertebral fractures in women with postmenopausal osteoporosis: a randomized controlled trial. JAMA. 1999;282:1344–52.
3. McClung MR, Geusens P, Miller PD, et al. Effect of risedronate on the risk of hip fracture in elderly women. N Engl J Med. 2001;344:333–40.
4. Chesnut CH III, Skag A, Christiansen C, et al. Effects of oral ibandronate administered daily or intermittently on fracture risk in postmenopausal osteoporosis. J Bone Miner Res. 2004;19:1241–9.
5. Black DM, Delmas PD, Eastell R, et al. Once-yearly zoledronic acid for treatment of postmenopausal osteoporosis. N Engl J Med. 2007;356:1809–22.
6. Cummings SR, San Martin J, McClung MR, et al. Denosumab for prevention of fractures in postmenopausal women with osteoporosis. N Engl J Med. 2009;361:756–65.
7. Tsourdi E, Langdahl B, Cohen-Solal M, et al. Discontinuation of denosumab therapy for osteoporosis: a systematic review and position statement by ECTS. Bone. 2017;105:11–7.

8. Ettinger B, Black DM, Mitlak BH, et al. Reduction of verte-bral fracture risk in postmenopausal women with osteoporosis treated with raloxifene: results from a 3-year randomized clinical trial. JAMA. 1999;282:637–45.

9. Silverman SL, Christiansen C, Genant HK, et al. Efficacy of bazedoxifene in reducing new vertebral fracture risk in post-menopausal women with osteoporosis: results from a 3-year, randomized, placebo-, and active-controlled clinical trial. J Bone Miner Res. 2008;23:1923–34.

10. Roelofs AJ, Thompson K, Gordon S, Rogers MJ. Molecular mechanisms of action of bisphosphonates: current status. Clin Cancer Res. 2006;12:6222s–30s.

11. Bone HG, Hosking D, Devogelaer JP, et al. Ten years' experience with alendronate for osteoporosis in postmenopausal women. N Engl J Med. 2004;350:1189–99.

12. Mellström DD, Sörensen OH, Goemaere S, Roux C, Johnson TD, Chines AA. Seven years of treatment with risedronate in women with postmenopausal osteoporosis. Calcif Tissue Int. 2004;75:462–8.

13. Black DM, Reid IR, Cauley JA, et al. The effect of 6 versus 9 years of zoledronic acid treatment in osteoporosis: a random-ized second extension to the HORIZON-Pivotal Fracture Trial (PFT). J Bone Miner Res. 2015;30:934–44.

14. Watts NB, Chines A, Olszynski WP, et al. Fracture risk remains reduced one year after discontinuation of risedronate. Osteoporos Int. 2008;19:365–72.

15. Black DM, Schwartz AV, Ensrud KE, et al. Effects of continuing or stopping alendronate after 5 years of treatment: the Fracture Intervention Trial Long-term Extension (FLEX): a randomized trial. JAMA. 2006;296:2927–38.

16. Black DM, Reid IR, Boonen S, et al. The effect of 3 versus 6 years of zoledronic acid treatment of osteoporosis: a random-ized extension to the HORIZON-Pivotal Fracture Trial (PFT). J Bone Miner Res. 2012;27:243–54.

17. McClung M, Harris ST, Miller PD, et al. Bisphosphonate therapy for osteoporosis: benefits, risks, and drug holiday. Am J Med. 2013;126:13–20.

18. Whitaker M, Guo J, Kehoe T, Benson G. Bisphosphonates for osteoporosis–where do we go from here? N Engl J Med. 2012;366:2048–51.

19. Rosen CJ, Brown S. Severe hypocalcemia after intravenous bisphosphonate therapy in occult vitamin D deficiency. N Engl J Med. 2003;348:1503–4.

20. Fosamax Prescribing Information. Merck & Co, Inc; 2012.
21. Actonal Prescribing Information. Warner-Chilcott US, LLC; 2015.
22. Reclast Prescribing Information. Novartis Pharmaceuticals Corp; 2015.
23. Lyles KW, Colón-Emeric CS, Magaziner JS, et al. Zoledronic acid and clinical fractures and mortality after hip fracture. N Engl J Med. 2007;357:1799–809.
24. Beaupre LA, Morrish DW, Hanley DA, et al. Oral bisphosphonates are associated with reduced mortality after hip fracture. Osteoporos Int. 2011;22:983–91.
25. Miller PD, Jamal SA, Evenepoel P, Eastell R, Boonen S. Renal safety in patients treated with bisphosphonates for osteoporosis: a review. J Bone Miner Res. 2013;28:2049–59.
26. Cummings SR, Eckert S, Krueger KA, et al. The effect of raloxifene on risk of breast cancer in postmenopausal women: results from the MORE randomized trial. JAMA. 1999;281:2189–97.
27. Evista Prescribing Information. Eli Lilly and Company; 2011.
28. Conbriza Prescribing Information [EMA]. Pfizer Limited; 2014.
29. Barrett-Connor E, Grady D, Sashegyi A, et al. Raloxifene and cardiovascular events in osteoporotic postmenopausal women: four-year results from the MORE randomized trial. JAMA. 2002;287:847–57.
30. McClung MR, Lewiecki EM, Cohen SB, et al. Denosumab in postmenopausal women with low bone mineral density. N Engl J Med. 2006;354:821–31.
31. Bone HG, Wagman RB, Brandi ML, et al. 10 years of denosumab treatment in postmenopausal women with osteoporosis: results from the phase 3 randomised FREEDOM trial and open-label extension. Lancet Diabetes Endocrinol. 2017;5:513–23.
32. Kendler DL, Roux C, Benhamou CL, et al. Effects of denosumab on bone mineral density and bone turnover in postmenopausal women transitioning from alendronate therapy. J Bone Miner Res. 2010;25:72–81.
33. Prolia Prescribing Information. Amgen Inc; 2017.
34. Jamal SA, Ljunggren O, Stehman-Breen C, et al. Effects of denosumab on fracture and bone mineral density by level of kidney function. J Bone Miner Res. 2011;26:1829–35.
35. Miller PD, Bolognese MA, Lewiecki EM, et al. Effect of denosumab on bone density and turnover in postmenopausal women with low bone mass after long-term continued, discontinued, and restarting of therapy: a randomized blinded phase 2 clinical trial. Bone. 2008;43:222–9.

36. Cummings SR, Ferrari S, Eastell R, et al. Vertebral fractures after discontinuation of denosumab: a post hoc analysis of the randomized placebo-controlled FREEDOM trial and its extension. J Bone Miner Res. 2018;33:190–8.
37. Neer RM, Arnaud CD, Zanchetta JR, et al. Effect of parathyroid hormone (1–34) on fractures and bone mineral density in postmenopausal women with osteoporosis. N Engl J Med. 2001;344:1434–41.
38. Keaveny TM, McClung MR, Wan X, Kopperdahl DL, Mitlak BH, Krohn K. Femoral strength in osteoporotic women treated with teriparatide or alendronate. Bone. 2012;50:165–70.
39. Forteo Prescribing Information. Eli Lilly and Company; 2012.
40. Kendler DL, Marin F, CAF Z, et al. Effects of teriparatide and risedronate on new fractures in post-menopausal women with severe osteoporosis (VERO): a multicentre, double-blind, double-dummy, randomised controlled trial. Lancet. 2017; pii: S0140-6736(17)32137-2

Chapter 6
Management of Patients with Increased Fracture Risk

Felicia Cosman

6.1 Introduction

Osteoporosis is often diagnosed in women and men in the sixth decade of life, resulting in up to 40 years during which bone loss progresses and fracture risk increases. Therefore, treatment decisions for osteoporosis should consider not just whether to treat but also what is the most rational approach to long-term control of the disease, with the goals of minimizing fracture risk while also minimizing risk of adverse events. Different medications are more appropriate at different ages and severity of the disease. Furthermore, proof of efficacy for any therapy beyond 5 years is limited, and some adverse events with potent anti-resorptive medication might be associated with duration of treatment. No osteoporosis medication should be used forever, and sequential monotherapy, rotating effective agents, is the most logical approach for most individuals.

F. Cosman (✉)
Helen Hayes Hospital, West Haverstraw, NY, USA
e-mail: christian.roux@cch.aphp.fr

© Springer Nature Switzerland AG 2019   59
S. L. Ferrari, C. Roux (eds.), *Pocket Reference to Osteoporosis*,
https://doi.org/10.1007/978-3-319-26757-9_6

This chapter provides a rationale for treatment decisions at different ages and stages of osteoporosis and discusses treatment sequences that are most likely to achieve the greatest therapeutic margin. The chapter will also cover a rationale for consideration of stopping therapy (and how to determine when and if to restart therapy). Finally, the chapter discusses the circumstances in which combination therapy should be considered.

6.2 Treatment for Younger Women (Early 50s to Mid or Late 60s) with Osteoporosis by Bone Mineral Density But No Fractures

Most logical for this group of women is a hormone regimen or tissue-selective estrogen complex (TSEC; conjugated estrogen/bazedoxifene), especially in women with active hot flashes, or an estrogen agonist/antagonist agent (EAA; raloxifene) in women without active hot flashes. Fracture risk in these younger individuals is low (especially in the absence of a history of fractures), and hip fracture is particularly rare [1]. Although younger individuals with a bone mineral density (BMD) diagnosis of osteoporosis have substantial lifelong risk, the short-term risk (over the ensuing decade) is in fact low. The major fractures of concern are vertebrae and wrist in this age group. All therapies, including hormone and EAA regimens, maintain and/or increase BMD and reduce risk of vertebral fractures [2–4]. Hormone therapy (HT) or TSEC therapies can be followed sequentially by an EAA in some individuals, once hot flashes and night sweats are no longer an issue, without worry about long-term adverse events in the skeleton. Furthermore, breast cancer risk reduction is an added benefit of EAA use [5]. If patients have fractures, lose bone, or simply reach an age where HT/estrogen therapy (ET), TSEC, and EAA therapies are no longer desirable (based on other risks such as venous thrombosis), a switch to more potent bone-specific anti-resorptive therapies should be considered (see below). Furthermore, fracture risk, including hip fracture risk, increases with age, so agents with known efficacy against fractures throughout the skeleton, and specifically the hip (see Chap. 5), would be required for most individuals with osteoporosis in their 70s and beyond.

6.3   Treatment for Older Women (Late 60s and Beyond) with Osteoporosis by Bone Mineral Density or an Isolated Fracture (Especially if More Remote)

As patients age, agents with efficacy across the skeleton (beyond the spine only), including TPTD, oral and i.v. bisphosphonates, and/or denosumab, are required. In older women with a recent hip fracture, yearly infusions of zoledronic acid have been demonstrated to reduce the incidence of second clinical fractures and to reduce mortality [6]. Denosumab may be preferable to bisphosphonates for patients who require more substantial increments in BMD, since with denosumab, BMD continues to increase in both the spine and hip after the first 3 years of treatment [7], whereas BMD plateaus in patients taking bisphosphonates after 3 years [8]. Therefore, patients with low BMD are more likely to achieve BMD goals (T-score at least > -2.5) when taking long-term denosumab compared with bisphosphonates.

6.4   Patients with Severe Osteoporosis at High Risk for Fractures

Anabolic therapy (i.e., teriparatide, TPTD, or abaloparatide) should be considered for patients who are at high risk of fracture (highest risk is in those patients with multiple fractures [9] and/or recent fractures [10–13]). Although anabolic therapy is more expensive than other therapies, the concept that it should be used only after "failing" a previous therapy is not logical. The only data that confirm efficacy against fractures are from patients who had not been on prior osteoporosis therapy [14]. Furthermore, in high-risk patients, teriparatide reduces fractures significantly compared to risedronate over a period of 24 months [12]. Patients who are transitioned from bisphosphonates or denosumab to TPTD or PTH have different BMD and bone turnover marker responses compared with treatment-naive patients [10, 11, 14–20]. This is particularly problematic for the hip and likely to be problematic in other cortical-predominant sites. Total hip and femoral neck BMD levels actually decline during the first year after the transition from bisphosphonates (alendronate and risedronate) or denosumab (where the decline is particularly marked) [21]. For patients who are being switched to anabolic therapy because of a recent fracture, declining BMD, or a stable but persistently low BMD, a decline in hip BMD is obviously not a desirable outcome. It is in these patients that combination therapy has the greatest potential.

6.5   Combination Therapy

Combination therapy with two anti-resorptive drugs is not justified. Although it is infrequently used, combination of an anti-resorptive with a bone-forming agent has some rationale. Combination therapy was formally tested in 102 women on prior alendronate who were randomized to continue or stop their anti-resorptive when TPTD was initiated [22]. This study was therefore a direct randomized comparison of TPTD monotherapy versus TPTD combination therapy in treatment-experienced patients. Although an anabolic response was seen, both biochemically and densitometrically in all groups, there was a greater increase in all biochemical turnover markers in those randomized to TPTD monotherapy. Of particular note was the early increase in the bone resorption marker, cross-linked C-telopeptide (CTX), which was already significantly elevated at 1 month in the patients assigned to TPTD monotherapy, suggesting that withdrawal of bisphosphonates results in exaggerated bone resorption upon exposure to TPTD. As a result, BMD declined in the first 6 months in the hip (consistent with all TPTD or PTH monotherapy studies in bisphosphonate-experienced patients). The BMD increments at both 6 and 18 months in both the spine and hip were greater in those patients randomized to the TPTD/alendronate combination compared with TPTD monotherapy, and at no time point did hip BMD decline in the combination therapy group [23]. This trial also formally evaluated a cohort of women on prior raloxifene treatment randomized to a TPTD/raloxifene combination versus TPTD monotherapy. Differences in BMD accrual were minimal between these groups.

Consistent with the DXA findings in patients on prior alendronate, volumetric BMD of the hip did not change in women who switched from alendronate to TPTD monotherapy but increased significantly at both 6 and 18 months in those who received combination TPTD/alendronate [24]. Furthermore, volumetric BMD of the cortical compartment of the hip declined significantly in those randomized to TPTD monotherapy. Strength of the hip, assessed by finite element analysis, did not decline with TPTD monotherapy implying that the decline in cortical BMD was not in an area critical for strength. However, hip strength increased significantly only with combination therapy.

Similar observations were made from a group of patients who were transitioned from denosumab (after 2 years) to TPTD. However, the effect of the transition from denosumab to TPTD monotherapy on hip BMD was far more prominent compared with the transition from bisphosphonates to TPTD [21]. Combination therapy has not been formally tested in women on prior denosumab (where TPTD is later added), but combination denosumab/TPTD has been investigated in women who were treatment-naive. In these patients, both spine and hip BMD increased more in the combination group than TPTD monotherapy, especially in the first year [25]. By analogy, this combination might be more effective than TPTD monotherapy in those previously treated with denosumab.

The findings from these studies have important implications for the clinical use of TPTD in patients who have received prior bisphosphonates or denosumab and are at high risk for fractures of the hip and other skeletal sites that are rich in cortical bone (e.g., a patient on bisphosphonate or denosumab who sustains a hip fracture). It may be that the withdrawal of the bisphosphonate or denosumab actually facilitates an exaggerated bone resorption response to TPTD and offsets the expected positive bone balance, particularly in the cortical skeleton, creating cortical porosity. In this case continuing the anti-resorptive while adding the bone-forming agent may therefore be a better option. The lack of substantial impact of prior raloxifene use on the subsequent use of TPTD is also important clinically because it provides a rationale for the use of raloxifene (and likely other EAA and TSEC agents) as a bridge to maintain BMD in younger patients who may need TPTD or abaloparatide later in life.

There are relatively few indications for combination therapy in patients who have not been on prior potent anti-resorptive treatment. Patients with recent hip and vertebral fractures could be considered for combination treatment with TPTD and denosumab. If this path is chosen, after combination treatment for up to 2 years, denosumab should be continued until BMD goals are achieved and patients remain free of fracture (at least for several years, including no new vertebral fractures documented by repeat spine imaging). Denosumab is also probably the agent of choice after treatment with TPTD monotherapy until BMD goals (T-score above −2.5) are achieved.

6.6   When Is Stopping Osteoporosis Treatment Reasonable?

BMD on osteoporosis therapy is a predictor of future fracture risk, just as BMD predicts fracture risk in treatment-naive individuals. Three large-scale osteoporosis treatment studies confirm this relationship. Two were randomized extensions of large pivotal fracture trials with alendronate and zoledronic acid [8, 26, 27], and one is an observational study of long-term use of denosumab [7]. These studies show that future fracture risk is dependent on the hip BMD level achieved during treatment. Those patients who still have osteoporosis after an initial treatment period have a future fracture risk similar to those with that BMD who have not yet been treated. This suggests that hip BMD above osteoporosis range (T-score > −2.5) should be a goal of osteoporosis therapy. It is critical to realize, however, that when non-bisphosphonate osteoporosis medications are stopped bone density declines quickly. This is true of all estrogen-containing agents, TPTD (and presumably abaloparatide), and denosumab. Moreover the rapid loss of bone mass after discontinuation of a medication such as denosumab is associated with structural deterioration and an increase in risk of (multiple) vertebral fractures [28]. Therefore, it is inadvisable to stop these agents. Non-bisphosphonate medications must be continued, or switched to a bisphosphonate, at least temporarily [29]. Because of the residual persistent effect of bisphosphonates after treatment discontinuation, therapy can be stopped after bisphosphonate use. During the off-treatment period after use of a bisphosphonate, maintenance of BMD or a much slower BMD loss after discontinuation can be expected (compared with all non-bisphosphonate compounds) [30, 31].

Therefore, it is possible to use non-bisphosphonate therapies to achieve a BMD target and then switch to bisphosphonate treatment to help maintain BMD. Patients who have not had recent fractures and who have BMD above the osteoporosis range, especially in the absence of multiple prevalent vertebral fractures, after 3–5 years of osteoporosis therapy or therapy sequences, are good candidates for temporary cessation of treatment. Table 6.1 provides a summary of the overall principles concerning switching and stopping osteoporosis medications.

TABLE 6.1 Key principles of stopping and switching osteoporosis medication

Key principles: stopping and switching osteoporosis medications

Stopping osteoporosis medications:

BMD loss will occur after stopping any non-bisphosphonate medications:

Most rapid loss occurs after stopping denosumab

BMD is maintained or lost slowly after stopping BPs:

BMD loss may be more rapid after stopping risedronate versus other BPs

BMD most likely to remain stable for several years after stopping zoledronic acid

If medication withdrawal is desirable after treatment with a non-bisphosphonate medication (especially denosumab, TPTD, or abaloparatide), switch to BP first, preferably zoledronic acid, for at least 1 year

Switches that are advisable:

From HT to EAA

From HT or EAAs to any other agent (TPTD/abaloparatide, denosumab, or BP).

From denosumab to BP

From BP to denosumab is ok but may increase BMD less than sequence of denosumab first followed by BP

From TPTD/abaloparatide to denosumab or BP

Switches that are not optimal:

From BP to TPTD/abaloparatide – expect some hip BMD loss or at least no gain for up to 18 months

From denosumab to TPTD/abaloparatide – expect dramatic hip BMD loss

BMD bone mineral density, *BP* bisphosphonate, *EAA* estrogen agonist/antagonist agent, *HT* hormone therapy, *PTH* parathyroid hormone, *TPTD* teriparatide

6.7   Resumption of Treatment After Medication Holiday

There is variability among the BPs regarding the duration of action after cessation of therapy (risedronate probably has the shortest and zoledronic acid probably has the longest duration of action) and substantial interindividual variability as well. Serum biochemical markers (yearly) and BMD (at least every 2 years) can be used to help determine when the effect of the bisphosphonate is diminishing. There is no evidence base upon which to make decisions about treatment resumption. Clinical logic suggests that a new fracture and/or a decline in BMD (greater than 4–5% which represents least significant change for BMD and a BMD T-score that is now again at ≤-2.5) would be a rationale for resumption of treatment. An increase in biochemical marker level more than double the nadir level and resulting in a level in the upper normal premenopausal range might also be a rationale for resuming osteoporosis treatment or at least watching BMD closely (maybe annually) as this marker level might be a sign of incipient active bone loss.

After a medication holiday, if treatment resumption is required, similar principles can be used regarding the selection of best medications or medication sequences as were used to select initial therapy.

6.8   Conclusion

When osteoporosis treatment is initiated, long-term treatment plans should be considered. Sequential monotherapy, rotating agents, is the best approach for most patients. Treatment sequence is of critical importance to maximize benefit and minimize risk. In general, anabolic agents should be used prior to potent anti-resorptive agents, and the latter should be reserved for individuals in their late 60s and beyond.

References

1. Harvey N, Dennison E, Cooper C. The epidemiology of osteoporotic fractures. In: Rosen CJ, editor. Primer on the metabolic bone diseases and disorders of mineral metabolism. 8th ed. UK: Wiley-Blackwell; 2013. p. 348–56.
2. Ettinger B, Black DM, Mitlak BH, Knickerbocker RK, Nickelsen T, Genant HK, et al. Reduction of vertebral fracture risk in postmenopausal women with osteoporosis treated with raloxifene: results from

a 3-year randomized clinical trial. Multiple Outcomes of Raloxifene Evaluation (MORE) Investigators. JAMA. 1999;282(7):637–45.

3. Rossouw JE, Anderson GL, Prentice RL, LaCroix AZ, Kooperberg C, Stefanick ML, et al. Risks and benefits of estrogen plus progestin in healthy postmenopausal women: principal results from the Women's Health Initiative randomized controlled trial. JAMA. 2002;288(3):321–33.

4. Cummings SR, Ensrud K, Delmas PD, LaCroix AZ, Vukicevic S, Reid DM, et al. Lasofoxifene in postmenopausal women with osteoporosis. N Engl J Med. 2010;362(8):686–96.

5. Vogel VG, Costantino JP, Wickerham DL, Cronin WM, Cecchini RS, Atkins JN, et al. Update of the National Surgical Adjuvant Breast and Bowel Project Study of Tamoxifen and Raloxifene (STAR) P-2 Trial: Preventing breast cancer. Cancer Prev Res (Phila). 2010;3(6):696–706.

6. Lyles KW, Colon-Emeric CS, Magaziner JS, Adachi JD, Pieper CF, Mautalen C, et al. Zoledronic acid and clinical fractures and mortality after hip fracture. N Engl J Med. 2007;357(18):1799–809.

7. Ferrari S, Adachi JD, Lippuner K, Zapalowski C, Miller PD, Reginster JY, et al. Further reductions in nonvertebral fracture rate with long-term denosumab treatment in the FREEDOM open-label extension and influence of hip bone mineral density after 3 years. Osteoporos Int. 2015;26(12):2763–71.

8. Black DM, Reid IR, Boonen S, Bucci-Rechtweg C, Cauley JA, Cosman F, et al. The effect of 3 versus 6 years of zoledronic acid treatment of osteoporosis: a randomized extension to the HORIZON-Pivotal Fracture Trial (PFT). J Bone Miner Res. 2012;27(2):243–54.

9. Gehlbach S, Saag KG, Adachi JD, Hooven FH, Flahive J, Boonen S, et al. Previous fractures at multiple sites increase the risk for subsequent fractures: the Global Longitudinal Study of Osteoporosis in Women. J Bone Miner Res. 2012;27(3):645–53.

10. Schousboe JT, Fink HA, Lui LY, Taylor BC, Ensrud KE. Association between prior non-spine non-hip fractures or prevalent radiographic vertebral deformities known to be at least 10 years old and incident hip fracture. J Bone Miner Res. 2006;21(10):1557–64.

11. van Geel TA, Huntjens KM, van den Bergh JP, Dinant G-J, Geusens PP. Timing of subsequent fractures after an initial fracture. Curr Osteoporos Rep. 2010;8(3):118–22.

12. Kendler DL, Marin F, Zerbini CA, Russo LA, Greenspan SL, Zikan V, et al. Effects of teriparatide and risedronate on new

fractures in post-menopausal women with severe osteoporosis (VERO): a multicentre, double-blind, double-dummy, randomised controlled trial. Lancet. 2018;391(10117):230–40.

13. Cosman F, de Beur SJ, LeBoff MS, Lewiecki EM, Tanner B, Randall S, et al. Clinician's guide to prevention and treatment of osteoporosis. Osteoporos Int. 2014;25(10):2359–81.

14. Cosman F. Combination therapy for osteoporosis: a reappraisal. BoneKEy Rep. 2014;3:518.

15. Lindsay R, Silverman SL, Cooper C, Hanley DA, Barton I, Broy SB, et al. Risk of new vertebral fracture in the year following a fracture. JAMA. 2001;285(3):320–3.

16. Johnell O, Kanis JA, Oden A, Sernbo I, Redlund-Johnell I, Petterson C, et al. Fracture risk following an osteoporotic fracture. Osteoporos Int. 2004;15(3):175–9.

17. Huntjens KM, Kosar S, van Geel TA, Geusens PP, Willems P, Kessels A, et al. Risk of subsequent fracture and mortality within 5 years after a non-vertebral fracture. Osteoporos Int. 2010;21(12):2075–82.

18. Center JR, Bliuc D, Nguyen TV, Eisman JA. Risk of subsequent fracture after low-trauma fracture in men and women. JAMA. 2007;297(4):387–94.

19. Cosman F, Nieves JW, Dempster DW. Treatment sequence matters: anabolic and antiresorptive therapy for osteoporosis. J Bone Miner Res. 2017;32(2):198–202.

20. Cosman F. Anabolic and antiresorptive therapy for osteoporosis: combination and sequential approaches. Curr Osteoporos Rep. 2014;12(4):385–95.

21. Leder BZ, Tsai JN, Uihlein AV, Wallace PM, Lee H, Neer RM, et al. Denosumab and teriparatide transitions in postmenopausal osteoporosis (the DATA-Switch study): extension of a randomised controlled trial. Lancet. 2015; 386(9999):1147–55.

22. Bone HG, Wagman RB, Brandi ML, Brown JP, Chapurlat R, Cummings SR, et al. 10 years of denosumab treatment in post-menopausal women with osteoporosis: results from the phase 3 randomised FREEDOM trial and open-label extension. Lancet Diabetes Endocrinol. 2017;5(7):513–23.

23. Cosman F, Wermers RA, Recknor C, Mauck KF, Xie L, Glass EV, et al. Effects of teriparatide in postmenopausal women with osteoporosis on prior alendronate or raloxifene: differences between stopping and continuing the antiresorptive agent. J Clin Endocrinol Metab. 2009;94(10):3772–80.

24. Cosman F, Keaveny TM, Kopperdahl D, Wermers RA, Wan X, Krohn KD, et al. Hip and spine strength effects of adding versus switching to teriparatide in postmenopausal women with osteoporosis treated with prior alendronate or raloxifene. J Bone Miner Res. 2013;28(6):1328–36.

25. Tsai JN, Uihlein AV, Lee H, Kumbhani R, Siwila-Sackman E, McKay EA, et al. Teriparatide and denosumab, alone or combined, in women with postmenopausal osteoporosis: the DATA study randomised trial. Lancet. 2013;382(9886):50–6.

26. Black DM, Schwartz AV, Ensrud KE, Cauley JA, Levis S, Quandt SA, et al. Effects of continuing or stopping alendronate after 5 years of treatment: the Fracture Intervention Trial Long-term Extension (FLEX): a randomized trial. JAMA. 2006;296(24):2927–38.

27. Cosman F, Cauley JA, Eastell R, Boonen S, Palermo L, Reid IR, et al. Reassessment of fracture risk in women after 3 years of treatment with zoledronic acid: when is it reasonable to discontinue treatment? J Clin Endocrinol Metab. 2014;99(12):4546–54.

28. Brown JP, Roux C, Torring O, Ho PR, Beck Jensen JE, Gilchrist N, et al. Discontinuation of denosumab and associated fracture incidence: analysis from the Fracture Reduction Evaluation of Denosumab in Osteoporosis Every 6 Months (FREEDOM) trial. J Bone Miner Res. 2013;28(4):746–52.

29. Freemantle N, Satram-Hoang S, Tang ET, Kaur P, Macarios D, Siddhanti S, et al. Final results of the DAPS (Denosumab Adherence Preference Satisfaction) study: a 24-month, randomized, crossover comparison with alendronate in postmenopausal women. Osteoporos Int. 2012;23(1):317–26.

30. Boonen S, Ferrari S, Miller PD, Eriksen EF, Sambrook PN, Compston J, et al. Postmenopausal osteoporosis treatment with antiresorptives: effects of discontinuation or long-term continuation on bone turnover and fracture risk--a perspective. J Bone Miner Res. 2012;27(5):963–74.

31. Reid IR, Black DM, Eastell R, Bucci-Rechtweg C, Su G, Hue TF, et al. Reduction in the risk of clinical fractures after a single dose of zoledronic Acid 5 milligrams. J Clin Endocrinol Metab. 2013;98(2):557–63.

Chapter 7
Management of Male Osteoporosis

Piet Geusens and Joop van den Bergh

7.1 Introduction

After middle age, osteoporosis-related fractures are more common in women than in men [1]. As a result, fracture prevention has been most extensively studied in postmenopausal women. However, between 30% and 40% of fractures due to osteoporosis occur in men, and the lifetime risk of fracture for men aged 50 or older is between 13% and 30% [2–4]. During aging, fracture risk rises exponentially in both sexes, but the increase occurs about a decade later in men than in women [1].

The mortality rate of patients with hip fractures older than 70 years is two to three times higher in men than in women [1]. In contrast to the risk of a first fracture after the age of 50 years, which is higher in women than in men, the risk of a subsequent fracture after a first fracture is the same for both sexes [5]. Therefore, men older than 50 years deserve attention for fracture risk evaluation and fracture prevention in high-risk patients.

P. Geusens (✉) · J. van den Bergh
Department of Internal Medicine, Maastricht University Medical Center, Maastricht, The Netherlands
e-mail: piet.geusens@scarlet.be

© Springer Nature Switzerland AG 2019
S. L. Ferrari, C. Roux (eds.), *Pocket Reference to Osteoporosis*,
https://doi.org/10.1007/978-3-319-26757-9_7

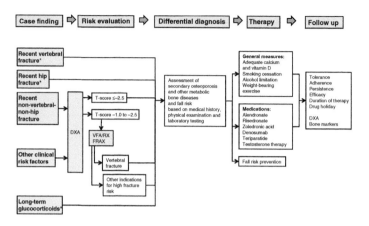

FIGURE 7.1 Fracture prevention algorithm in men: a five-step decision plan. In green, recommendations according to Watts et al. [9]. *DXA not strictly necessary for therapeutic decisions, but helpful for follow-up. (Adapted from Ref. [9])

Fracture prevention consists of a systematic multistep approach that starts with clinical case finding, followed by evaluation, differential diagnosis, treatment, and follow-up [6]. There is a wealth of evidence for the efficacy of each of these steps in women, but the evidence for efficacy in men is less well documented. As a result, most of the current fracture prevention guidelines are for women at high risk of fractures [7].

Fracture prevention can be summarized in a five-step evaluation and treatment plan as presented in Fig. 7.1 based on recommendations from the American Endocrine Society review in 2012 [8, 9] and a review paper of a European expert panel in 2013 [10].

7.2   Case Finding

The first step is clinical case finding, which means that men at risk for future fractures should be recognized. We propose two patient risk profiles: men older than 50 years with a history of fracture after 50 years of age and men with no history of fractures but with clinical risk factors for fracture [9].

7.2.1 Men with a History of Fracture

In men with a history of fracture, the risk of subsequent fractures is increased and is highest in the first years after a fracture. Evaluation of fracture risk and underlying diseases is therefore advocated as soon as possible after a recent fragility fracture. In this context, the fracture liaison service (FLS) with a specialized osteoporosis nurse under supervision of a specialist (surgeon, endocrinologist, rheumatologist, geriatrician) is considered as the most effective case finding strategy [11, 12].

7.2.2 Men Without a History of Fracture

In men without a history of fracture, clinical case finding takes into account age, body mass index (BMI), parent with hip fracture, a fall in the past year, inability to complete a walking test, diseases/conditions related to loss of bone mineral density (BMD), or increased risk of fractures such as delayed puberty, hypogonadism, hyperparathyroidism, hyperthyroidism, chronic obstructive pulmonary disease, drugs such as glucocorticoids or GnRH agonists, and lifestyle choices such as alcohol abuse and smoking [9, 13].

7.3 Risk Evaluation

To evaluate fracture risk, clinical risk factors, assessment of BMD using dual-energy X-ray absorptiometry (DXA), and imaging of the spine by radiography or vertebral fracture assessment (VFA) using DXA technology are available. VFA has the advantage of low radiation dose, and it has a high negative predictive value [14].

7.3.1 Men with a History of Fracture

The presence of a low-trauma vertebral or hip fracture is generally considered a sufficiently high risk of subsequent fractures for pharmaceutical treatment to be recommended without the requirement for using DXA. However, a baseline DXA and imaging of the full spine may be useful for decision-making during follow-up.

In men with a non-vertebral non-hip fracture, measurement of BMD using DXA is recommended, and if osteoporosis is diagnosed (T-score ≤ −2.5), pharmacological treatment should be initiated. VFA and prediction of fracture risk using the Fracture Risk Assessment (FRAX®) calculator are recommended for men with a non-vertebral non-hip fracture and osteopenia (T-score between −1 and −2.5). In these men, pharmacological treatment is recommended if a vertebral fracture is present or, in the USA, if the FRAX risk for major fractures is ≥20% and/or the FRAX risk for hip fracture is ≥3% [9]. In a European expert review, it was stated that treatment is widely recommended in men after any fragility fracture [10].

7.3.2   Men Without a History of Fracture

In men older than 70 years, measurement of BMD using DXA is suggested, whereas in men aged 50–69 years, DXA of the spine and hip is suggested if fracture risk factors are present. Fracture risk calculators such as FRAX® (www.shef.ac.uk) and the Garvan fracture risk calculator (www.garvan.org.au) can aid patient evaluation.

Treatment is advocated if the patient has osteoporosis or osteopenia, if VFA indicates the presence of a previously undiagnosed vertebral fracture, or, in the USA, if the patient's 10-year FRAX risk is ≥20% for major fractures or ≥3% for hip fracture. Regardless of DXA result, pharmaceutical treatment is recommended for men who receive ≥7.5 mg/day long-term prednisone or an equivalent glucocorticoid therapy.

7.4   Differential Diagnosis

The next step in the evaluation and treatment plan is the differential diagnosis. A complete history and physical examination is suggested for men who are being evaluated for osteoporosis or considered for pharmacological treatment. The aim is to gather information regarding evidence of causes of secondary osteoporosis or other metabolic bone diseases, fall risk, and overall frailty. Laboratory evaluation with measurement of serum calcium, phosphate, creatinine (with estimated glomerular filtration rate), alkaline phosphatase, liver function, 25hydroxyvitamin D, total testosterone, thyroid-stimulating hormone (TSH), complete blood count, and 24hour urinary calcium (creatinine and sodium) excretion is suggested [9, 15]. Additional laboratory testing should be carried out if the patient's medical history or the results of the physical examination suggest a specific cause of osteoporosis. Such testing might include, but is not limited to, analysis of the level of sex hormone-binding globulin, tissue transglutaminase antibodies (for diagnosis of celiac disease) or parathyroid hormone, serum protein electrophoresis (with free κ and λ light chains) and/or urine protein electrophoresis, and additional thyroid function tests [9, 15].

7.5   Treatment

Following differential diagnosis, treatment should be initiated in men at high risk of fracture. A daily total calcium intake of 1000–1200 mg and cessation of smoking are recommended, and weight-bearing exercises, limiting alcohol intake to <3 units/day, and vitamin D supplementation (if serum levels are <75 nmol/l) are suggested for men with, or at increased risk of, osteoporosis and fractures [9].

Regulatory agencies accept studies for reimbursement when surrogate endpoints, such as changes in BMD, are comparable to changes that are attained in women (in studies with fracture endpoint). The antiresorptive drugs alendronate [16, 17], risedronate [18], ibandronate [19], zoledronic acid [20–22], strontium ranelate [23], and denosumab [24, 25] have been investigated in male populations with low BMD. All studies had BMD as the primary endpoint and demonstrated a significant BMD increase [16–25]. In terms of BMD, zoledronic acid was not inferior compared to alendronate but also not superior [20]. Strontium ranelate increases BMD as in women [23], but its mechanism of action is still unclear [26]. Two studies reported fracture reduction as a secondary outcome [16, 18]. In other studies, the number of fractures was too small to allow for statistical analyses.

Only one intervention study with reduction of vertebral fractures as primary endpoint is available in men: zoledronic acid significantly reduced the risk of vertebral fractures compared with placebo (primary endpoint) [22]. In the study by Lyles et al. [21], a post recent hip fracture study, zoledronic acid decreased second subsequent clinical fractures in a population with both males and females by 35% and mortality from any cause by 28%. Therefore, treatment with zoledronate is suggested for men with a recent hip fracture [9].

In men receiving androgen deprivation therapy for nonmetastatic prostate cancer, denosumab was associated with a reduction in the incidence of new vertebral fractures [27] and is recommended for men with prostate cancer who are receiving androgen deprivation therapy [9].

Teriparatide increased BMD in men compared with placebo [28, 29], and men who received teriparatide and who may have received follow-up antiresorptive therapy had a decreased risk of moderate and severe vertebral fractures [30].

Initiation of testosterone therapy instead of anti-osteoporosis medication is suggested for men with a borderline high risk of fracture who have serum testosterone levels <6.9 nmol/l on more than one determination and signs or symptoms of androgen deficiency. Testosterone therapy is also suggested for men at high risk of fracture with testosterone levels <6.9 nmol/l who lack standard indications for testosterone therapy but have contraindications to approved pharmacological agents for osteoporosis [9]. An agent with proven anti-fracture efficacy, such as a bisphosphonate or teriparatide, is suggested for men at high risk of fracture who are receiving testosterone therapy [9].

7.6   Follow-Up

The final stage of the evaluation and treatment plan is follow-up to evaluate tolerance, adherence, persistence, and efficacy of therapy and to decide about duration of therapy, drug holiday, and switching of therapy. Monitoring BMD using DXA of the spine and hip, bone resorption markers, such as levels of serum Ctelopeptide or urine Ntelopeptide of type I collagen, can be used to monitor antiresorptive therapy responses, and bone formation markers, such as serum procollagen I Npropeptide, can be used to monitor responses to anabolic therapy. However, appropriate values for bone markers to indicate optimal response to treatment remain unclear [9]. No studies are available on the duration of treatment and eventual drug holiday. A man of 75 years of age with a fracture still has a mean lifetime expectancy of 8 years; thus long-term treatment decisions are necessary [31]. As proposed in women, re-evaluation after 5-year therapy using clinical risk factors and DXA would allow physicians to identify patients at low fracture risk (e.g., BMD above a T-score of −1.0 or −2.5), in whom treatment could be temporarily interrupted, and patients at high risk, in whom treatment should continue [32].

7.7   Conclusion

Based on the available literature, recommendations for multi-step fracture prevention in men can be formulated [8, 9]. However, high-quality evidence is not available to support any of the recommendations or suggestions. Further studies are, therefore, required to increase the level of evidence for optimal fracture prevention in men to a level comparable to that in women. In the context of gendered medicine and innovations, fracture prevention in men deserves more attention [33].

References

1. Johnell O, Kanis JA. An estimate of the worldwide prevalence and disability associated with osteoporotic fractures. Osteoporos Int. 2006;17:1726–33.
2. Cooper C, Melton LJ 3rd. Epidemiology of osteoporosis. Trends Endocrinol Metab. 1992;3:224–9.

3. Bliuc D, Nguyen ND, Milch VE, Nguyen TV, Eisman JA, Center JR. Mortality risk associated with low-trauma osteoporotic fracture and subsequent fracture in men and women. JAMA. 2009;301:513–21.

4. van Helden S, van Geel AC, Geusens PP, Kessels A, Nieuwenhuijzen Kruseman AC, Brink PR. Bone and fall-related fracture risks in women and men with a recent clinical fracture. J Bone Joint Surg Am. 2008;90:241–8.

5. van Geel TA, van Helden S, Geusens PP, Winkens B, Dinant GJ. Clinical subsequent fractures cluster in time after first fractures. Ann Rheum Dis. 2009;68:99–102.

6. van den Bergh JP, van Geel TA, Geusens PP. Osteoporosis, frailty and fracture: implications for case finding and therapy. Nat Rev Rheumatol. 2012;8:163–72.

7. Leslie WD, Schousboe JT. A review of osteoporosis diagnosis and treatment options in new and recently updated guidelines on case finding around the world. Curr Osteoporos Rep. 2011;9:129–40.

8. Geusens PP, Bone v d BJP. New guidelines for multistep fracture prevention in men. Nat Rev Rheumatol. 2012;8:568–70.

9. Watts NB, Adler RA, Bilezikian JP, et al. Osteoporosis in men: an Endocrine Society clinical practice guideline. J Clin Endocrinol Metab. 2012;97:1802–22.

10. Kaufman JM, Reginster JY, Boonen S, et al. Treatment of osteoporosis in men. Bone. 2013;53:134–44.

11. Akesson K, Marsh D, Mitchell PJ, et al. Capture the fracture: a best practice framework and global campaign to break the fragility fracture cycle. Osteoporos Int. 2013;24:2135–52.

12. McLellan AR, Gallacher SJ, Fraser M, McQuillian C. The fracture liaison service: success of a program for the evaluation and management of patients with osteoporotic fracture. Osteoporos Int. 2003;14:1028–34.

13. Lewis CE, Ewing SK, Taylor BC, et al. Predictors of non-spine fracture in elderly men: the MrOS study. J Bone Miner Res. 2007;22:211–9.

14. Chapurlat RD, Duboeuf F, Marion-Audibert HO, Kalpakcioglu B, Mitlak BH, Delmas PD. Effectiveness of instant vertebral assessment to detect prevalent vertebral fracture. Osteoporos Int. 2006;17:1189–95.

15. Bours SP, van den Bergh JP, van Geel TA, Geusens PP. Secondary osteoporosis and metabolic bone disease in patients 50 years and

older with osteoporosis or with a recent clinical fracture: a clinical perspective. Curr Opin Rheumatol. 2014;26:430–9.

16. Orwoll E, Ettinger M, Weiss S, et al. Alendronate for the treatment of osteoporosis in men. N Engl J Med. 2000;343:604–10.

17. Gonnelli S, Cepollaro C, Montagnani A, et al. Alendronate treatment in men with primary osteoporosis: a three-year longitudinal study. Calcif Tissue Int. 2003;73:133–9.

18. Boonen S, Orwoll ES, Wenderoth D, Stoner KJ, Eusebio R, Delmas PD. Once-weekly risedronate in men with osteoporosis: results of a 2-year, placebo-controlled, double-blind, multicenter study. J Bone Miner Res. 2009;24:719–25.

19. Orwoll ES, Binkley NC, Lewiecki EM, Gruntmanis U, Fries MA, Dasic G. Efficacy and safety of monthly ibandronate in men with low bone density. Bone. 2010;46:970–6.

20. Orwoll ES, Miller PD, Adachi JD, et al. Efficacy and safety of a once-yearly i.v. Infusion of zoledronic acid 5 mg versus a once-weekly 70-mg oral alendronate in the treatment of male osteoporosis: a randomized, multicenter, double-blind, active-controlled study. J Bone Miner Res. 2010;25:2239–50.

21. Lyles KW, Colon-Emeric CS, Magaziner JS, et al. Zoledronic acid and clinical fractures and mortality after hip fracture. N Engl J Med. 2007;357:1799–809.

22. Boonen S, Reginster JY, Kaufman JM, et al. Fracture risk and zoledronic acid therapy in men with osteoporosis. N Engl J Med. 2012;367:1714–23.

23. Kaufman JM, Audran M, Bianchi G, et al. Efficacy and safety of strontium ranelate in the treatment of osteoporosis in men. J Clin Endocrinol Metab. 2013;98:592–601.

24. Orwoll E, Teglbjaerg CS, Langdahl BL, et al. A randomized, placebo-controlled study of the effects of denosumab for the treatment of men with low bone mineral density. J Clin Endocrinol Metab. 2012;97:3161–9.

25. Langdahl BL, Teglbjaerg CS, Ho PR, et al. A 24-month study evaluating the efficacy and safety of denosumab for the treatment of men with low bone mineral density: results from the ADAMO trial. J Clin Endocrinol Metab. 2015;100:1335–42.

26. Chavassieux P, Meunier PJ, Roux JP, Portero-Muzy N, Pierre M, Chapurlat R. Bone histomorphometry of transiliac paired bone biopsies after 6 or 12 months of treatment with oral strontium ranelate in 387 osteoporotic women: randomized comparison to alendronate. J Bone Miner Res. 2014;29:618–28.

27. Smith MR, Egerdie B, Hernandez Toriz N, et al. Denosumab in men receiving androgen-deprivation therapy for prostate cancer. N Engl J Med. 2009;361:745–55.

28. Orwoll ES, Scheele WH, Paul S, et al. The effect of teriparatide [human parathyroid hormone (1-34)] therapy on bone density in men with osteoporosis. J Bone Miner Res. 2003;18:9–17.

29. Kurland ES, Cosman F, McMahon DJ, Rosen CJ, Lindsay R, Bilezikian JP. Parathyroid hormone as a therapy for idiopathic osteoporosis in men: effects on bone mineral density and bone markers. J Clin Endocrinol Metab. 2000;85:3069–76.

30. Kaufman JM, Orwoll E, Goemaere S, et al. Teriparatide effects on vertebral fractures and bone mineral density in men with osteoporosis: treatment and discontinuation of therapy. Osteoporos Int. 2005;16:510–6.

31. Abrahamsen B, Osmond C, Cooper C. Life expectancy in patients treated for osteoporosis: observational cohort study using national Danish prescription data. J Bone Miner Res. 2015;30:1553–9.

32. McClung M, Harris ST, Miller PD, et al. Bisphosphonate therapy for osteoporosis: benefits, risks, and drug holiday. Am J Med. 2013;126:13–20.

33. Schiebinger L, Klinge I, Sánchez de Madariaga I, Paik HY, Schraudner M, Stefanick M (eds). Osteoporosis research in men: rethinking standards and reference models. Gendered Innovations in Science, Health & Medicine, Engineering and Environment (2011–2015). https://genderedinnovations.stanford.edu/case-studies/osteoporosis.html. Accessed 14 Jan 2016.

Chapter 8
Management of Glucocorticoid-Induced Osteoporosis

Christian Roux

8.1 Introduction

Glucocorticoid-induced osteoporosis (GIOP) is the most common cause of secondary osteoporosis, the first cause before 50 years, and the first iatrogenic cause of the disease. There is a huge variability of side effects of glucocorticoids (GCs) among individuals for largely unknown reasons. However, in the context of the use of GCs, bone fragility is characterized by the rapidity of bone loss and the occurrence of fractures within the first months of use of GCs, indicating the need for appropriate early management of the patients.

The main effect of the use of GCs on bone is the impairment in bone formation, related to the decrease in osteoblast differentiation, the increase in osteoblast and osteocyte apoptosis, and the anti-anabolic effects such as a decrease in insulin-like growth factor 1 (IGF1) [1]. This reduced bone formation occurs in a situation of abnormal bone turnover:

C. Roux (✉)
Department of Rheumatology, Paris Descartes University, Cochin Hospital, Paris, Paris, France
e-mail: christian.roux@aphp.fr

© Springer Nature Switzerland AG 2019
S. L. Ferrari, C. Roux (eds.), *Pocket Reference to Osteoporosis*,
https://doi.org/10.1007/978-3-319-26757-9_8

inflammation by itself is responsible for enhanced osteoclastogenesis and osteoclast activity through the production of receptor activator of nuclear factor-kappaB (RANK) ligand by activated lymphocytes. Expression of sclerostin (inhibitor of formation) is also increased in models of inflammation. Thus, the introduction of GCs is associated with an uncoupling between high bone resorption and low bone formation [2]. Taking GCs also has indirect effects of reduced production of sexual steroids and myopathy and muscle weakness, responsible in turn for an increased risk of falls.

8.2   Fracture Risk

The risk of fractures is increased twofold in patients receiving GCs and is even higher for vertebral fractures (VFs). Asymptomatic VFs are frequent in patients receiving long-term GCs because of the analgesic effect of the treatment. Patient height must be measured at the initiation of GCs, and height loss must be checked in the follow-up for diagnosis of incident vertebral fractures. The increase in risk is immediate and occurs as early as 3 months after the initiation of therapy; thus primary prevention is highly recommended.

The assessment of fracture risk [3] is based on:

- Classical risk factors of osteoporosis – age, female gender, low body mass index, history of falls, previous fractures, duration of menopause, and smoking.
- Characteristics of GC therapy – the risk is mainly associated with recent and prolonged GC use rather than remote and short-term use.
- Characteristics of the underlying inflammatory disease including the potential previous deleterious effect of chronic inflammation.

Thus the Fracture Risk Assessment (FRAX) tool may help in GIOP, in order to take into account the whole list of risk factors. Adjustment of FRAX has been proposed for postmenopausal women and men aged ≥50 years with lower or higher doses than 2.5–7.5 mg/day: a factor of 0.8 for low-dose exposure and 1.15 for high-dose exposure for major osteoporotic fractures and 0.65 and 1.20 for hip fracture probability. For very high doses of GCs, greater upward adjustment of fracture probability may be required.

The interpretation of bone mineral density (BMD) is difficult in patients with GC treatment, as there is an unmatched data between BMD and fracture data. BMD can be normal and the bone fragility being high, because of alteration of bone quality. The threshold (in T-score) below which patients with GCs are at risk is unknown. A practical approach is to consider that a low BMD at the initiation of GCs, or underlying osteoporosis, is by itself a strong risk factor for immediate fractures.

8.3 Management of Patients with Glucocorticoid-Induced Osteoporosis

The first step for treatment is to review the daily dose of GCs. Physicians should consider reducing the dose to the lowest active dose, the use of immunosuppressive drugs as GCs sparing agents, and local (i.e., intra-articular) administration of the treatment.

The second step is the use of anti-osteoporotic treatment such as bisphosphonates, denosumab, and teriparatide, which have been assessed in both the prevention and treatment of GIOP. At the initiation of GCs, bisphosphonates (alendronate, risedronate, and zoledronate) prevent the bone loss, which in contrast is observed in the placebo groups (although appropriately treated by calcium and vitamin D). These drugs can increase BMD in patients with established GIOP. The efficacy on fractures is not a direct evidence from studies; it is mainly based on bridging data between the short-term change in BMD in patients with GCs and the long-term change in BMD and reduction of fracture risk in patients with postmenopausal osteoporosis.

Teriparatide is the first-choice therapy in patients with established GIOP, as the principal cause of bone fragility is reduction in bone formation. Moreover, in a prospective comparative study, the use of teriparatide was associated with fewer VFs than the use of alendronate.

There are a number of guidelines on the use of pharmacological treatment in GIOP, published by different national societies and colleges, which vary somewhat [4, 5]. However, all of them stress the early increase in the risk of fracture at the initiation of GCs and the importance of recognition of patients at high risk of fracture. For such patients (elderly subjects, patients who already have osteoporosis, and patients on high doses of GCs), primary prevention is always recommended.

There is no recommendation for the duration of treatment in GIOP. It must be prolonged if an individual has underlying osteoporosis and other risk factors for osteoporosis. Whether the treatment can be stopped in some individuals with normal BMD, absence of prevalent fractures, and quiescent underlying inflammatory disease is a research question.

References

1. Canalis E, Mazziotti G, Giustina A, Bilezikian JP. Glucocorticoid-induced osteoporosis: pathophysiology and therapy. Osteoporos Int. 2007;18:1319–28.
2. Roux C. Osteoporosis in inflammatory joint diseases. Osteoporos Int. 2011;22:421–33.
3. van Staa TP, Geusens P, Bijlsma JW, Leufkens HG, Cooper C. Clinical assessment of the long-term risk of fracture in patients with rheumatoid arthritis. Arthritis Rheum. 2006;54:3104–12.
4. Grossman JM, Gordon R, Ranganath VK, et al. American College of Rheumatology 2010 recommendations for the prevention and treatment of glucocorticoid-induced osteoporosis. Arthritis Care Res (Hoboken). 2010;62:1515–26.
5. Lekamwasam S, Adachi JD, Agnusdei D, et al. A framework for the development of guidelines for the management of glucocorticoid-induced osteoporosis. Osteoporos Int. 2012;23:2257–76.

Chapter 9
New Bone-Forming Agents

Socrates E. Papapoulos

9.1 Introduction

Pharmacological interventions for patients with osteoporosis aim at decreasing the risk of fractures and associated clinical consequences by correcting the imbalance between bone resorption and bone formation that constitutes the pathophysiological basis of the disease. Despite the availability of efficacious treatments for fracture reduction, there are still unmet needs requiring a broader range of therapeutics. In particular, there is a need for agents capable of replacing already lost bone and of drastically reducing the risk of nonvertebral fractures, the most frequent fragility fractures. In recent years, new molecules and therapeutic targets have been identified, and many were investigated as potential treatments for osteoporosis [1]. This chapter briefly reviews newly developed bone-forming agents.

S. E. Papapoulos (✉)
Center for Bone Quality, Leiden University Medical Center, Leiden, The Netherlands
e-mail: s.e.papapoulos@lumc.nl

© Springer Nature Switzerland AG 2019
S. L. Ferrari, C. Roux (eds.), *Pocket Reference to Osteoporosis*,
https://doi.org/10.1007/978-3-319-26757-9_9

9.2   Parathyroid Hormone-Related Peptides

Parathyroid hormone (PTH) peptides (e.g., teriparatide) bind to PTH/PTHrP type 1 receptor (PTH1R) in osteoblasts and osteocytes and stimulate bone formation but also bone resorption in patients with osteoporosis [2]. PTHrP, a protein with homology to PTH at the amino terminus that also binds to PTHR1, was hypothesized to increase bone formation with less increase in bone resorption than teriparatide making it an attractive bone-forming treatment for osteoporosis. Abaloparatide, a novel 34 aa synthetic peptide analog of PTHrP given by daily sc injections, increased BMD at the spine and the hip, in the latter at a level significantly higher than teriparatide (Fig. 9.1). In addition, abaloparatide increased biochemical markers of bone formation and resorption to a lesser extent than teriparatide despite being administered at a higher dose (80 μg/d vs 20 μg/d) [3].

The efficacy of abaloparatide in the prevention of fractures was evaluated in a phase III clinical trial of 2463 women with osteoporosis randomized to receive abaloparatide

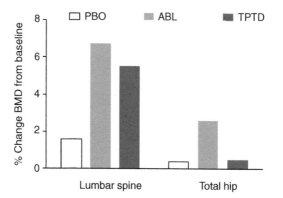

FIGURE 9.1 Percentage changes of bone mineral density (BMD) of postmenopausal women with osteoporosis after 24 weeks of treatment with subcutaneous injections of placebo (PBO), abaloparatide (ABL) 80 μg/d, and teriparatide (TPTD) 20 μg/d. (Adapted from Leder et al. [3])

80 µg/d sc, placebo sc, or open-label teriparatide 20 µg/d sc for 18 months [4]. Compared with placebo, abaloparatide reduced the risk of new vertebral fractures by 86% and of non-vertebral fractures by 43%; the decreases with teriparatide were 80% and 28% (ns), respectively. Abaloparatide was well tolerated – the most frequently reported adverse events were back pain, arthralgia, upper respiratory tract infection, hypercalciuria, and dizziness. The incidence of hypercalcemia 4 h after the injection was 0.37%, 3.41%, and 6.36% for the placebo, abaloparatide, and teriparatide groups, respectively.

9.3   Sclerostin Inhibitors

The role of sclerostin in bone metabolism was identified in studies of patients with sclerosteosis and van Buchem disease, two rare sclerosing bone dysplasias characterized by progressive generalized overgrowth and thickening of bone that is resistant to fracture. The two disorders are due to different defects of the SOST gene, located on chromosome 17q12–21, and result in impaired production of sclerostin. Sclerostin, a glycoprotein produced in the skeleton exclusively by osteocytes, is transported to the bone surface where it inhibits bone formation by antagonizing the canonical Wnt signaling pathway in osteoblasts [5, 6]; sclerostin also upregulates RANKL synthesis by osteocytes thereby stimulating osteoclastogenesis [7] (Fig. 9.2).

The restricted expression of sclerostin in the skeleton, and the lack of abnormalities in organs other than the skeleton in humans and animals with sclerostin deficiency, made this protein a target of new bone-building therapies for osteoporosis [9]. A number of sclerostin inhibitors have been investigated in preclinical and early clinical studies, but only one humanized monoclonal antibody, romosozumab, was tested in phase III clinical studies of women with postmenopausal osteoporosis. Romosozumab stimulated trabecular and cortical bone formation and increased bone mass and strength in animal models [10–12]. Importantly, the majority of new bone formation induced by romosozumab was modeling-based, occurring at quiescent surfaces, which is a clear anabolic

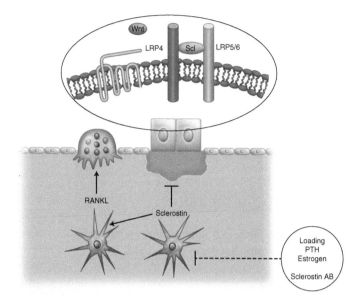

FIGURE 9.2 Schematic representation of sclerostin actions. Osteocyte-produced sclerostin inhibits the proliferation, differentiation, and survival of osteoblasts and reduces bone formation. It also stimulates the production of RANKL by neighboring osteocytes and bone resorption. In osteoblasts, sclerostin binds to LRP5/LRP6 and inhibits the Wnt signaling pathway, an action facilitated by LRP4. Production of sclerostin is decreased by mechanical loading, PTH, estrogens, and other factors. LRP4/LRP5/LRP6 low-density lipoprotein receptor-related protein 4/low density lipoprotein receptor-related protein 5/low density lipoprotein receptor-related protein 6, PTH parathyroid hormone, RANKL receptor activator of nuclear factor kappa-B ligand, Scl sclerostin. (Reproduced from Appelman-Dijkstra and Papapoulos [8])

response [13]. The effect of sclerostin inhibition on bone formation decreased with prolongation of treatment and was reversible upon its discontinuation.

Romosozumab given by monthly sc injections rapidly increased areal and volumetric BMD at the spine and the hip to levels clearly higher than daily teriparatide in treatment-naïve women as well as in osteoporotic women previously treated with bisphosphonate [14–17]. Adverse events were similar between placebo and romosozumab-treated patients with the exception of mild reactions at the injection sites [15]. Changes of biochemical markers and histological parameters of bone turnover in animals and humans during treatment with romosozumab were different from those observed during treatment with PTH or PTHrP peptides (Fig. 9.3) and suggested a functional uncoupling between bone formation and bone resorption.

There was an early rapid increase in bone formation followed by a progressive decline with time, which was not due to the development of neutralizing antibodies. The increase in bone formation was associated with a decrease of bone resorption, possibly through an inhibitory effect of the antibody on the production of RANKL by osteocytes. Treatment prolonging, however, appears to modestly reduce bone resorption but also bone turnover. It may thus be that while romosozumab acts as a pure anabolic agent in the beginning of treatment its

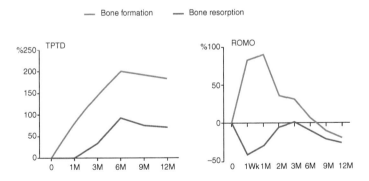

FIGURE 9.3 Schematic representation of changes in the levels of biochemical markers of bone turnover during treatment with subcutaneous injections of teriparatide (TPTD, 20 μg daily) or romosozumab (ROMO, 210 mg once monthly) for 1 year. Bone formation and bone resorption were assessed by measuring serum levels of procollagen type 1 aminoterminal propeptide (P1NP) and carboxyterminal collagen cross-linking (CTX), respectively. (Reproduced from Papapoulos [14])

continued administration results in mild inhibition of bone resorption and reduction of the remodeling space.

In one phase III clinical trial (FRAME) 7180 postmenopausal women aged between 55 and 90 years with BMD T-scores between −2.5 and −3.5 at the total hip or femoral neck were randomized to once-monthly sc injections of romosozumab (ROMO) 210 mg or placebo for 1 year followed by open-label denosumab (DMab) 60 mg sc every 6 months for a further 12 months; all women received vitamin D and calcium supplements [18]. Compared with placebo, ROMO treatment decreased the incidence of vertebral fractures by 73% at 12 months and by 75%, after transition to DMab, at 24 months. The risk of clinical fractures decreased significantly by 36% at 12 months while that of non-vertebral fractures by 25%, a nonsignificant result, probably due to lack of an effect in patients from Latin America with very low fracture risk. In study sites from the rest of the world, a 42% significant reduction in the incidence of non-vertebral fractures was observed. Adverse events, including serious cardiovascular events, osteoarthritis, and cancer, were balanced between the two groups. One case adjudicated as atypical femoral fracture was observed 3.5 months after the first ROMO injection in a patient with prodromal symptoms before starting treatment and two cases of osteonecrosis of the jaw after 12-month ROMO and 12-month ROMO and one dose DMab, respectively.

In the other phase III clinical trial (ARCH), 4039 women, mean age 74.3 years, with severe postmenopausal osteoporosis at high risk of fractures were randomized to receive sc ROMO 210 mg once monthly or oral alendronate (ALN) 70 mg once weekly for 12 months; thereafter, all patients received ALN until the end of the trial with maintenance of blinding to the initial treatment assignment; all women received daily calcium and vitamin D [19]. A superior anti-fracture efficacy of ROMO treatment was already evident at 12 months, and the incidence of all osteoporotic fractures, including those of the hip, decreased significantly in women treated with ROMO/ALN compared with those treated with ALN/ALN. Adverse events and serious adverse events were balanced between the two groups. However, during the first year of the study, positively adjudicated serious cardiovascular events were observed more often with ROMO than with ALN (50 vs 38 patients, respectively). Whether this imbalance was a chance finding, as it was not observed in the placebo-controlled FRAME study, or whether it was due to inhibition of sclerostin in the vasculature or to a protective effect of ALN need to be clarified [20]. During the second year of open-label ALN treatment two cases of osteonecrosis of the jaw (one in each group) and six cases of adjudicated atypical femoral fractures (two in the ROMO/ALN group and four in the ALN/ALN group) were observed.

The Wnt signaling pathway, a key regulator of bone formation, provided a number of targets for the development of bone anabolic therapies to fulfill an unmet need of patients with severe osteoporosis. Of these, sclerostin emerged as the preferred target due to its bone specificity and dual action on bone formation and resorption. Of the different sclerostin inhibitors developed, romosozumab was extensively investigated in adequately designed and performed preclinical and clinical studies. Results showed superior efficacy of romosozumab compared with existing therapies, and the magnitude of the rapid, pronounced gains of bone mass on treatment superseded those of other therapeutics. Thus, sclerostin inhibition met expectations of an efficacious anabolic therapy to fulfill a currently unmet need in the management of patients with severe osteoporosis. The imbalance, however, of serious cardiovascular events in the ARCH study, needs to be clarified.

9.4   Conclusion

The two components of bone remodeling resorption and formation constitute the primary target of pharmacological interventions for the management of the disease. It is now clear that bone resorption and formation can be differently modulated by new classes of anti-osteoporotic medications [8] that provide a novel, personalized perspective for the management of patients in clinical practice.

References

1. Appelman-Dijkstra NM, Papapoulos SE. Novel approaches to the treatment of osteoporosis. Best Pract Res Clin Endocrinol Metab. 2014;28:843–57.
2. Compston JE. Skeletal actions of intermittent parathyroid hormone: effects on bone remodelling and structure. Bone. 2007;40:1447–52.
3. Leder BZ, O'Dea LS, Zanchetta JR, et al. Effects of abaloparatide, a human parathyroid hormone-related peptide analog, on bone mineral density in postmenopausal women with osteoporosis. J Clin Endocrinol Metab. 2015;100:697–706.
4. Miller PD, Hattersly G, Riis BJ, et al. Effect of abaloparatide vs placebo on new vertebral fractures in postmenopausal women with osteoporosis: a randomized clinical trial. JAMA. 2016;316:722–33.
5. Moester MJ, Papapoulos SE, Lowik CW, van Bezooijen RL. Sclerostin: current knowledge and future perspectives. Calcif Tissue Int. 2010;87:99–107.
6. van Lierop AH, Appelman-Dijkstra NM, Papapoulos SE. Sclerostin deficiency in humans. Bone. 2017;96:51–62.
7. Wijenayaka AR, Kogawa M, Lim HP, Bonewald LF, Findlay DM, Atkins GJ. Sclerostin stimulates osteocyte support of osteoclast activity by a RANKL-dependent pathway. PLoS One. 2011;6:e25900.
8. Appelman-Dijkstra NM, Papapoulos SE. Modulating bone resorption and bone formation in opposite directions in the treatment of postmenopausal osteoporosis. Drugs. 2015;75:1049–58.
9. Appelman-Dijkstra NM, Papapoulos SE. Sclerostin inhibition in the management of osteoporosis. Calcif Tissue Int. 2016;98:370–80.
10. Li X, Warmington KS, Niu QT, et al. Inhibition of sclerostin by monoclonal antibody increases bone formation, bone mass, and bone strength in aged male rats. J Bone Miner Res. 2010;25:2647–56.
11. Ominsky MS, Vlasseros F, Jolette J, et al. Two doses of sclerostin antibody in cynomolgus monkeys increases bone formation, bone mineral density, and bone strength. J Bone Miner Res. 2010;25:948–59.
12. Ominsky MS, Boyce RW, Li X, Ke HZ. Effects of sclerostin antibodies in animal models of osteoporosis. Bone. 2017;96:63–75.

13. Ominsky MS, Niu QT, Li C, Li X, Ke HZ. Tissue-level mechanisms responsible for the increase in bone formation and bone volume by sclerostin antibody. J Bone Miner Res. 2014;29:1424–30.

14. Papapoulos SE. Anabolic bone therapies in 2014: new bone-forming treatments for osteoporosis. Nat Rev Endocrinol. 2015;11:69–70.

15. McClung MR, Grauer A, Boonen S, et al. Romosozumab in postmenopausal women with low bone mineral density. N Engl J Med. 2014;370:412–20.

16. Genant HK, Engelke K, Bolognese MA, et al. Effects of romosozumab compared with teriparatide on bone density and mass at the spine and hip in postmenopausal women with low bone mass. J Bone Miner Res. 2017;32:181–7.

17. Langdahl BL, Libanati C, Crittenden DB, et al. Romosozumab (sclerostin monoclonal antibody) versus teriparatide in postmenopausal women with osteoporosis transitioning from oral bisphosphonate therapy: a randomised, open-label, phase 3 trial. Lancet. 2017;390:1585–94.

18. Cosman F, Crittenden DB, Adachi JD, et al. Romosozumab treatment in postmenopausal women with osteoporosis. N Engl J Med. 2016;375:1532–43.

19. Saag KG, Petersen J, Brandi ML, et al. Romosozumab or alendronate for fracture prevention in women with osteoporosis. N Engl J Med. 2017;377:1417–27.

20. Appelman-Dijkstra NM, Papapoulos SE. Clinical advantages and disadvantages of anabolic bone therapies targeting the WNT pathway. Nat Rev Endocrinol. 2018;14:605–23.

Index

© Springer Nature Switzerland AG 2019
S. L. Ferrari, C. Roux (eds.), *Pocket Reference to Osteoporosis*,
https://doi.org/10.1007/978-3-319-26757-9